SUNNYBROOK HOSPITAL

SUNNYBROOK HOSPITAL

Our Veterans' Legacy of Care, a Photographic Journey Through the Decades

DR. PEETER A. POLDRE, EDITOR

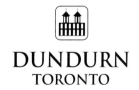

DUNDURN
TORONTO

Copy Editor: Cheryl Hawley
Design: Jennifer Scott
Printer: Friesens

Library and Archives Canada Cataloguing in Publication

Poldre, Peeter Antonio, 1953-
     Sunnybrook Hospital : our veterans' legacy of care, a photo journey through the decades / Peeter A. Poldre.

ISBN 978-1-55488-943-3

1. Sunnybrook Health Sciences Centre--History.   2. Sunnybrook Health Science Centre--Pictorial works.   3. Veterans' hospitals--Ontario--Toronto--History.   4. Veterans' hospitals--Ontario--Toronto--Pictorial works.   I. Title.

RA983.T62S86 2011   362.1109713'541   C2010-907736-9

1   2   3   4   5   15   14   13   12   11

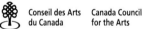 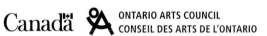

We acknowledge the support of the **Canada Council for the Arts** and the **Ontario Arts Council** for our publishing program. We also acknowledge the financial support of the **Government of Canada** through the **Canada Book Fund** and **Livres Canada Books**, and the **Government of Ontario** through the **Ontario Book Publishers Tax Credit** program, and the **Ontario Media Development Corporation**.

Care has been taken to trace the ownership of copyright material used in this book. The author and the publisher welcome any information enabling them to rectify any references or credits in subsequent editions.

J. Kirk Howard, President

Printed and bound in Canada.
www.dundurn.com

Dundurn Press
3 Church Street, Suite 500
Toronto, Ontario, Canada
M5E 1M2

Gazelle Book Services Limited
White Cross Mills
High Town, Lancaster, England
LA1 4XS

Dundurn Press
2250 Military Road
Tonawanda, NY
U.S.A. 14150

This book is dedicated to the war veterans at Sunnybrook, for whom the hospital was built, and to the caregivers — professional staff, volunteers, learners — who have honoured the contributions of our veterans by creating a legacy of internationally renowned patient care, education, and research.

The generosity of the Raab family has made it possible for us to share our veterans' legacy of care.

Contents

CHAPTER 1

The Sunnybrook History —
At the Beginning

THE HISTORY OF SUNNYBROOK HOSPITAL begins with two unrelated events early in the twentieth century.

In 1909, Joseph Kilgour, President of the Canada Paper Company, established one of Bayview Avenue's first country estates, south of Lawrence Avenue. He and his wife, Alice, named it Sunnybrook Farm. After Kilgour's death in 1928, the 178-acre property was donated to the city of Toronto by Alice, in memory of her husband. The intention was to retain it as parkland.

In 1919, to serve the needs of Canada's veterans returning from the Great War, the Toronto (Dominion) Military Orthopaedic Hospital was established on Christie Street, near Dupont Avenue, in a building that had formerly housed the National Cash Register Company. In 1936, the hospital was formally renamed the Christie Street Veterans Hospital.

As wounded veterans began returning from the Second World War there was significant public concern about the facilities on Christie Street. By 1942, the Greater Toronto Veterans Hospital Committee (chaired by the Honourable W.J. Stewart, CBE) spearheaded the initiative to build a new hospital for the veterans. The committee, and many other individuals, groups, and organizations, lobbied intensely. Sunnybrook Farm was ultimately identified as the preferred site. The heirs of the Kilgour estate approved. On August 10, 1943, Toronto Mayor Fred Conboy announced that the City of Toronto would provide the land (then Sunnybrook Park) to the Department of Veterans Affairs.

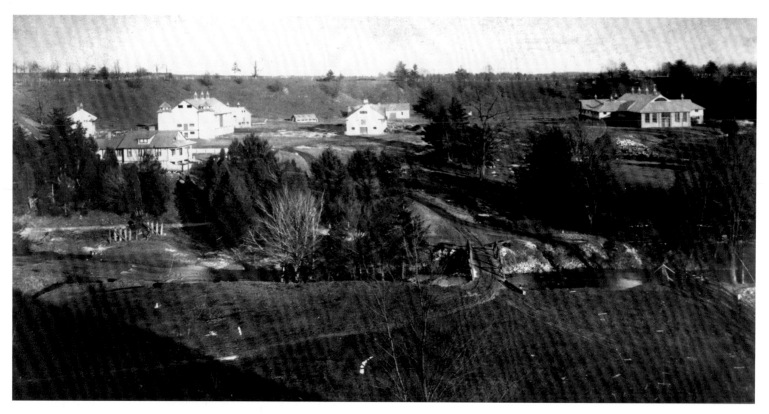

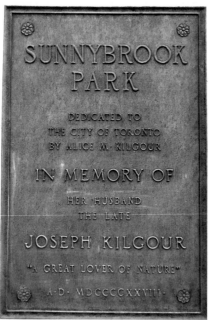

ABOVE: *Sunnybrook Farm (1910).*

LEFT: *Sunnybrook Park dedication plaque (1928).*

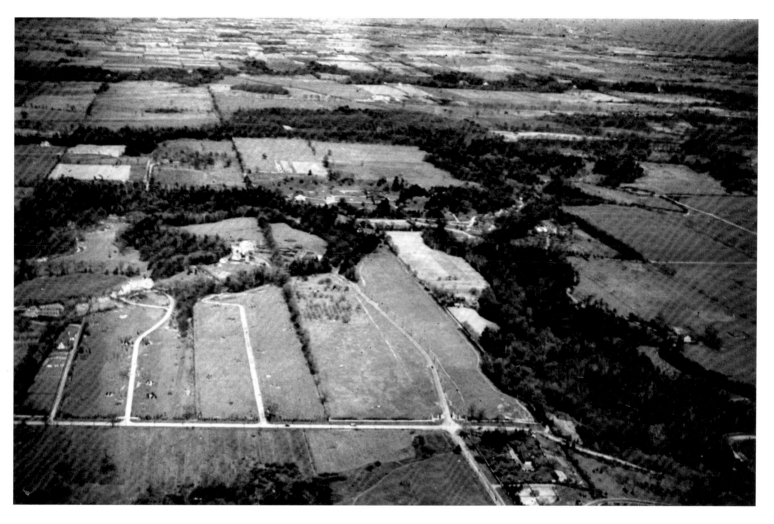

Aerial photo of Sunnybrook Park (c. 1940).

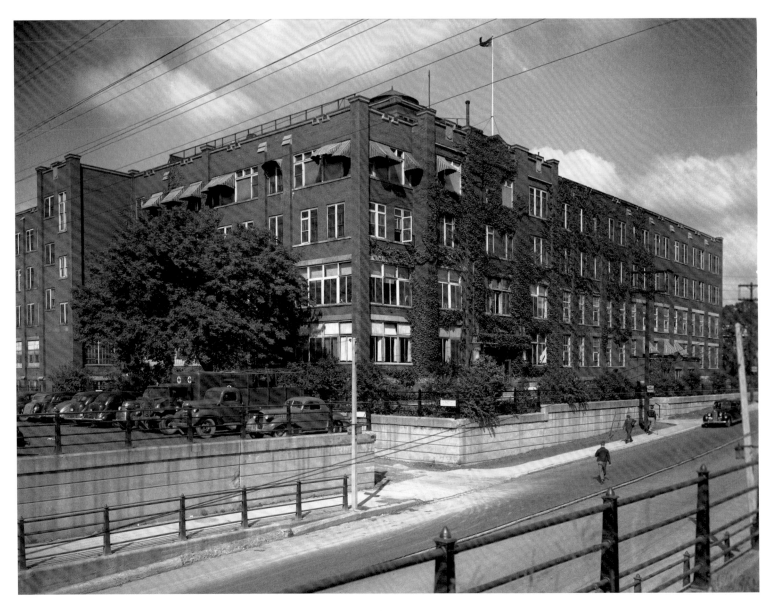

Christie Street Veterans Hospital (c. 1940).

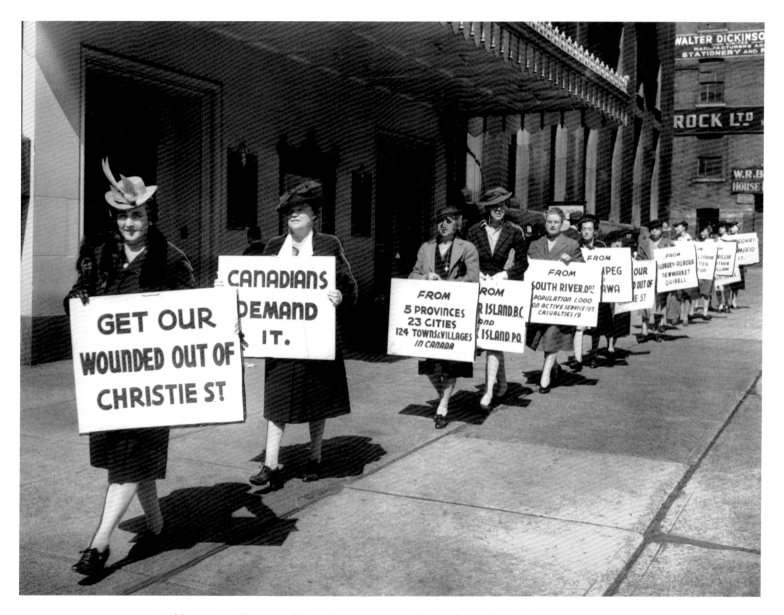

Public protest about conditions for veterans at Christie Street Hospital.
(Photo courtesy of the Globe and Mail*)*

Architects Allward and Gouinlock were commissioned to design the new hospital. On Remembrance Day 1943, the first sod was turned. On November 11, 1944, the Honourable Ian Mackenzie laid the cornerstone for the Neuropsychiatric Building. In June 1945, the Red Cross Lodge foundation stone was laid by the Honourable Leopold McCauley on the current site of the Odette Cancer Centre. (Today, that stone sits in front of the Veterans Centre as a tribute to all of the Red Cross volunteers who have cared for Canada's veterans over the years.) On November 11, 1945, Corporal Fred Topham, VC, laid the cornerstone for the Active Treatment Building of the hospital. In 1945, Dr. Karl E. Hollis was appointed as the first Hospital Superintendent.

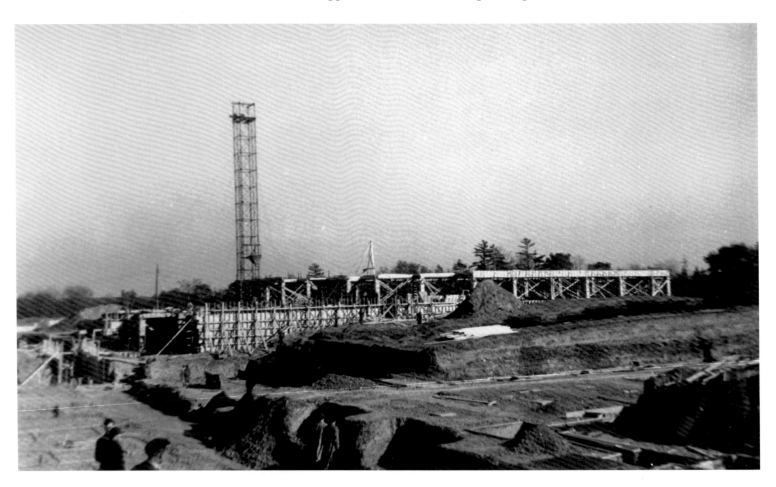

Sunnybrook Hospital construction (c. 1944).

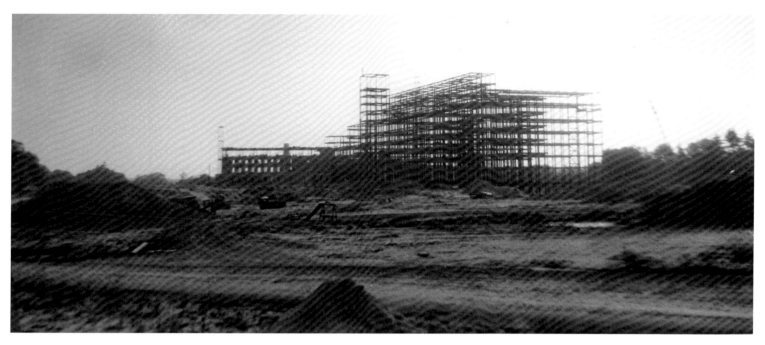

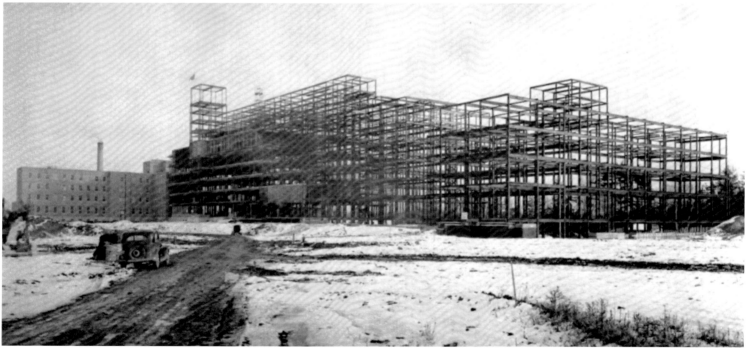

Sunnybrook Hospital construction.

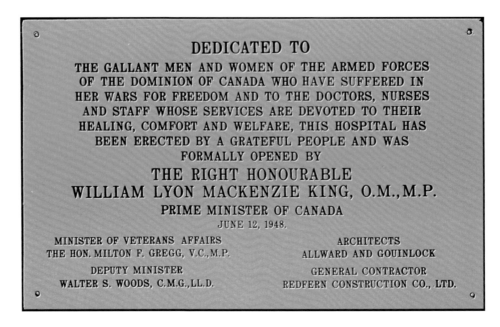

Plaque honouring the service of men and women of the armed forces and the medical staff at Sunnybrook.

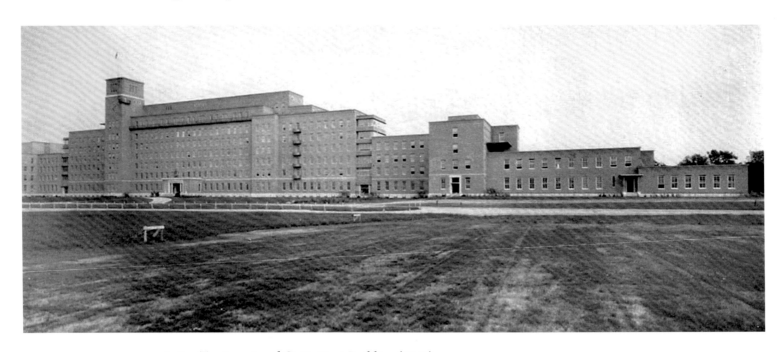

Active Treatment and Outpatient Building (1948).

On September 26, 1945, Private Raymond Scott was the first patient to enter Sunnybrook Hospital, as one of a group of 87 walking patients and 14 stretcher patients transferred from Christie Street Hospital. These first patients were located on D-Wing, named "Lancaster." Dr. William Baillie was the physician responsible for their care. Dr. "Casey" Little, who was in charge of medical services at Christie Street Hospital, oversaw the transfer and practised at Sunnybrook until he retired in 1952.

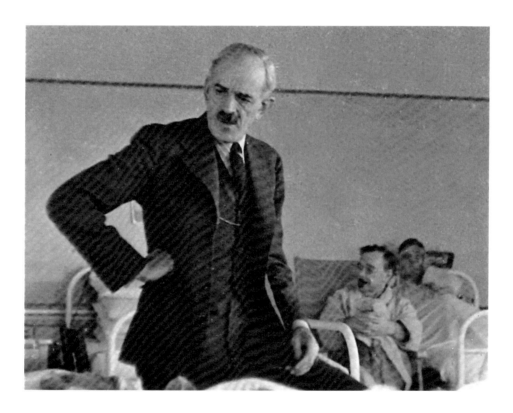

Dr. Oliver "Casey" Little with veterans at Christie Street Hospital.
(Photo courtesy of Derek Little)

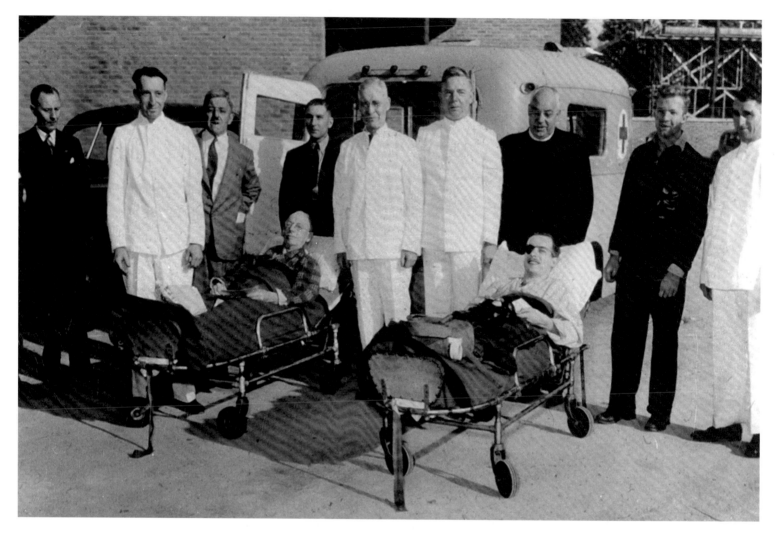

First veterans transferred from Christie Street to Sunnybrook (1945).

The Red Cross Lodge formally opened on January 30, 1947. Canadian Red Cross Society volunteers provided services and recreational activities to veterans at Sunnybrook until the year 2000.

Construction on the main building proceeded well and by early 1948 another 42 patients from Christie Street were admitted to C-Wing, named "Spitfire." Dr. Ian Macdonald, Sunnybrook's first Physician-in-Chief, was responsible for their care.

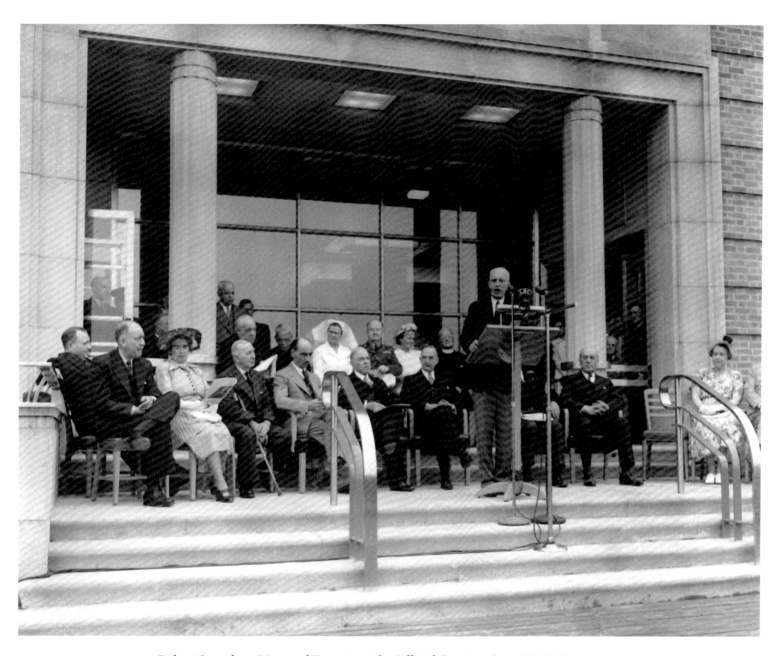

Robert Saunders, Mayor of Toronto, at the Official Opening, June 12, 1948.

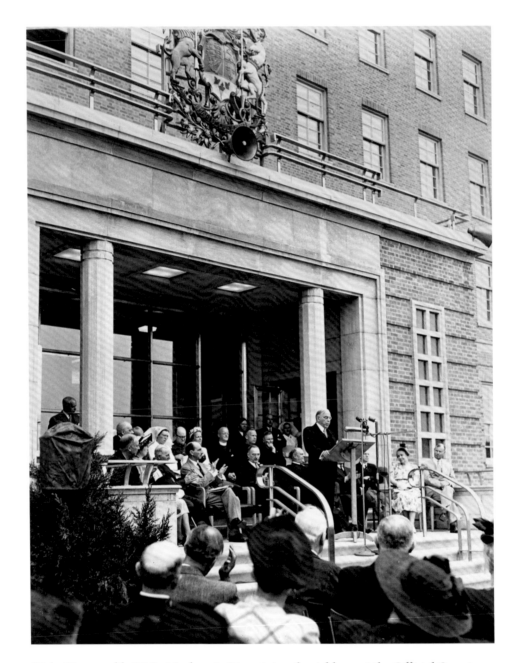

Right Honourable W. L. Mackenzie King giving the Address at the Official Opening, June 12, 1948.

In creating Sunnybrook Hospital, the Government of Canada sought to express the enduring gratitude felt by all Canadians to the veterans of Canada's wars and conflicts. The words inscribed on the Sunnybrook Cenotaph serve to illustrate this commitment: ***To honour the dead and to care for the sick and the injured Sunnybrook Hospital stands as a living memorial to the men and women of the Armed Forces of Canada.***

The provision of medical care and comfort to those who were maimed, disabled, or rendered infirm continues to the present.

Sunnybrook's official opening occurred on Saturday June 12, 1948. The Minister of Veterans Affairs, the Honourable Milton Gregg, VC, CBE, was introduced by W.J. Stewart, CBE.

The Prime Minister of Canada, the Right Honourable William Lyon Mackenzie King, OM, officially opened Sunnybrook Hospital,

> In Sunnybrook Hospital, the Government of Canada has sought to give some expression to the gratitude and obligations felt by all Canadians toward those veterans of the two great wars who were maimed, disabled or rendered infirm in the defence of freedom, and who are still in need of medical care and attention. As an institution of healing, this vast, modern hospital has received the highest praise from hospital authorities throughout the world. Sunnybrook Hospital symbolizes Canada's recognition of the sacrifices made by those members of the armed forces whom the hospital aims to serve, and seeks to honour.

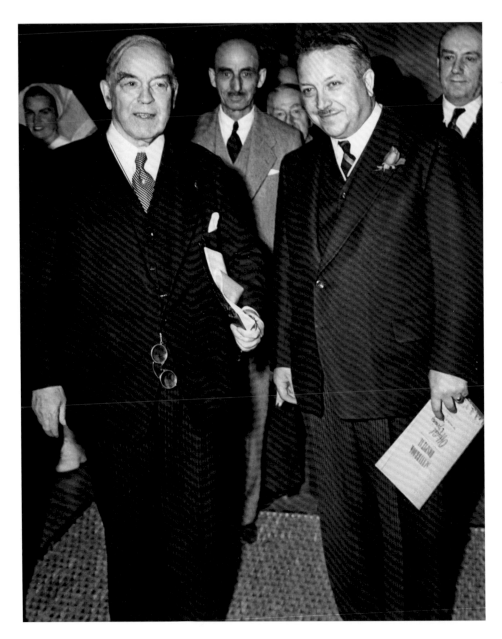

Right Honourable W. L. Mackenzie King with guests at the Official Opening,
June 12, 1948.

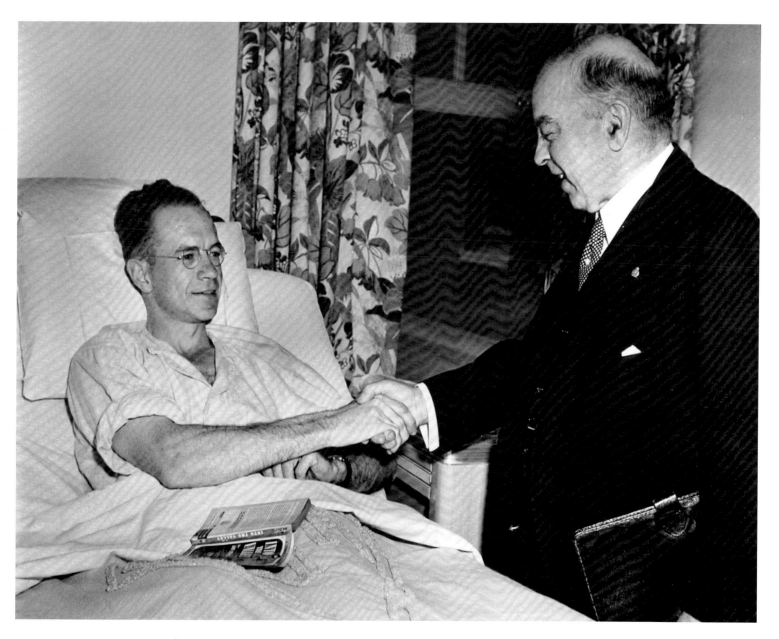

Right Honourable W. L. Mackenzie King visiting a veteran (June 12, 1948).

CHAPTER 2

Coming of Age (1948–1966)

AFTER THE OFFICIAL OPENING, THE hard work of living up to the expectations set by Prime Minister Mackenzie King began in earnest. Remembrances of the wars were everywhere. Early hospital wings were named in honour of the Canadian Army in the First World War (Ypres); the Canadian Army in the Second World War (Ortona and Falaise); the Canadian Navy (Atlantic); and the Canadian Air Force (Lancaster and Spitfire).

By 1950, Sunnybrook was truly a magnificent sight. The construction used 5.5 million bricks, 3,750 doors, 3,000 windows, 80 acres of plastering, 4,500 tons of cut stone, and piping for plumbing and heating that extended for 125 miles. In all, the hospital included 2,800 rooms. The floor area of the original hospital was approximately 21 acres. Designed for up to 1,600 patients, the hospital included an Outpatient Block, the Active Treatment Building, the Neuropsychiatry Building, and a maintenance and power plant. A nurses' residence, prosthetics building, chapel, therapeutic pool and gymnasium, and a large auditorium enhanced the building. Seven operating theatres in the Active Treatment Building were ultra-modern in construction and equipment and completely explosion-proof.

The interior décor in the new hospital was also created with care and artistry. William A. Howard was the chief interior designer, responsible for the fabrics, colour schemes, and furniture, much of which was specially crafted. Numerous beautiful murals graced several common areas of the hospital.

SUNNYBROOK HOSPITAL

The main entrance murals were the creation of Russian-born artists René and André Kulbach. Other murals, some still visible in room E110, were created by Eric Aldwinckle and Angus MacDonald.

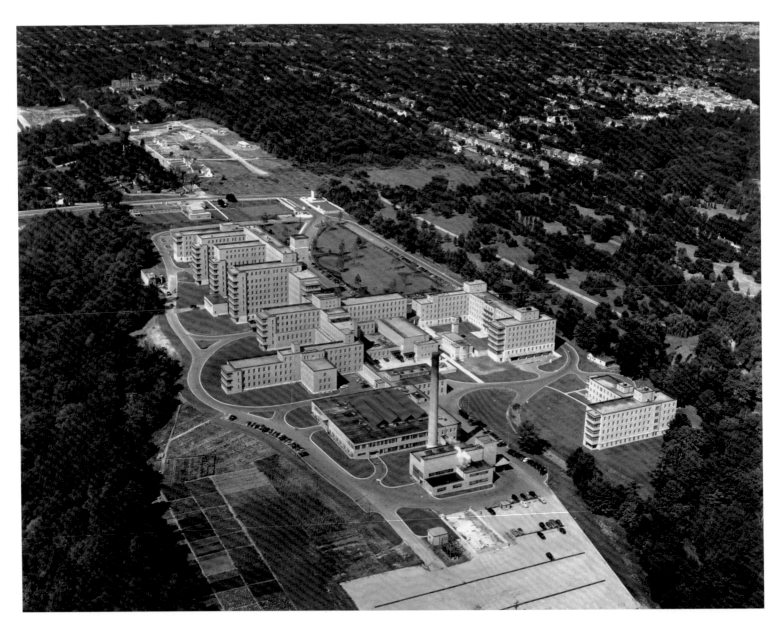

Aerial photo of Sunnybrook, from the east, showing the patients' garden (lower left).

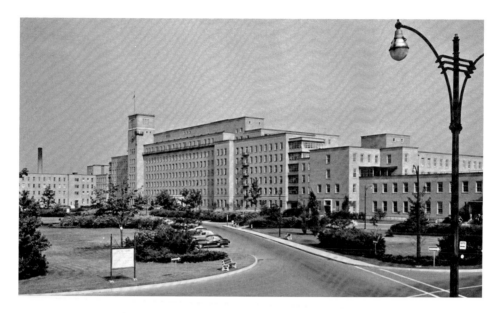

Main entrance to the Sunnybrook campus from Bayview Avenue.

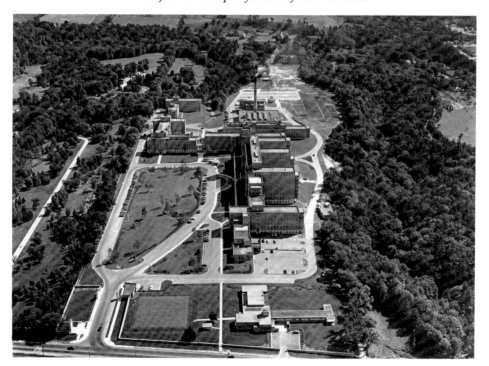

Aerial photo, from the west, with the Red Cross Lodge and the lawn bowling green at the bottom.

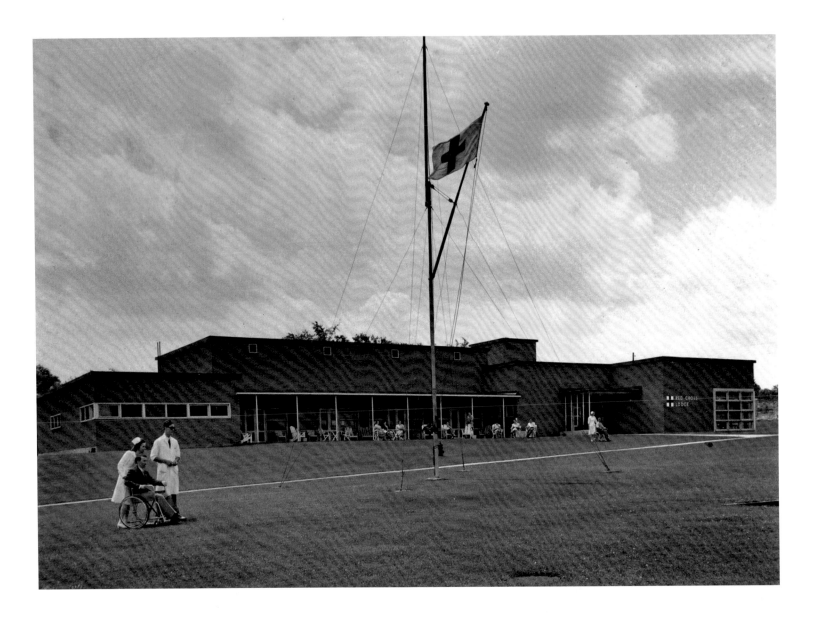

ABOVE: *Red Cross Lodge (c. 1948).*

FACING: *Playing shuffleboard in the basement of the Red Cross Lodge.*

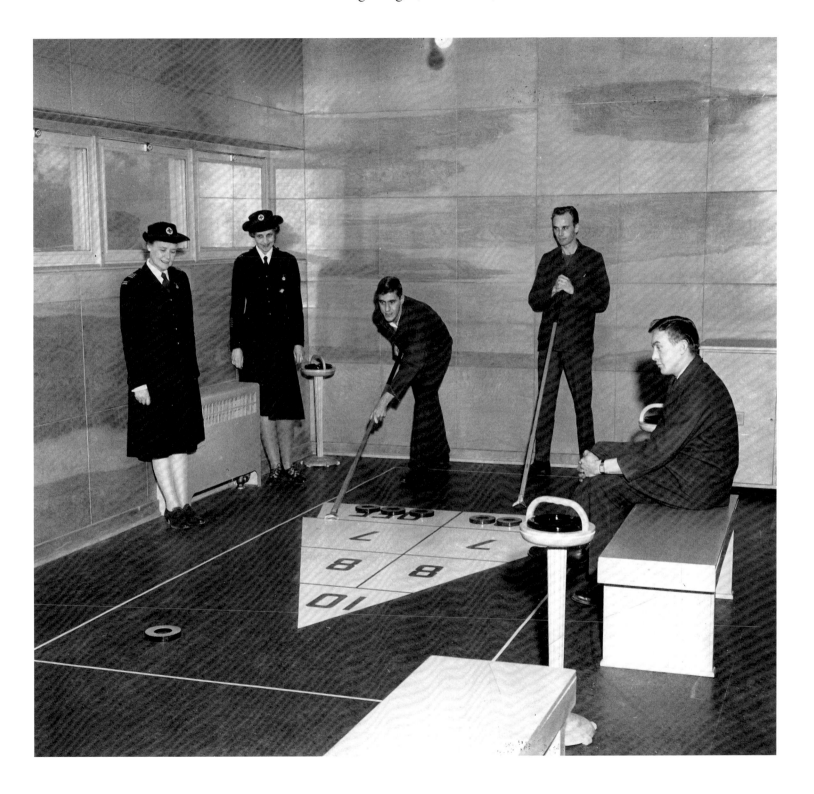

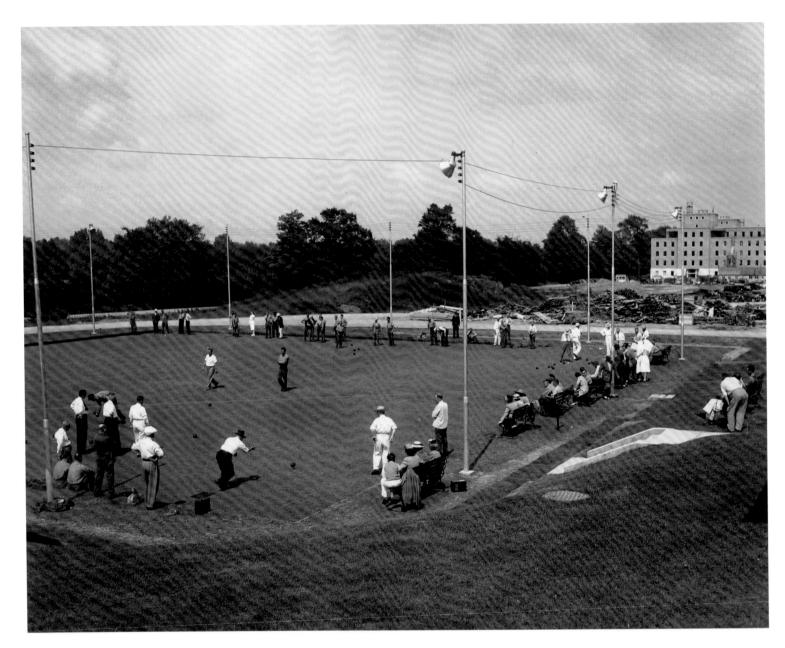

Lawn bowling in front of Red Cross Lodge.

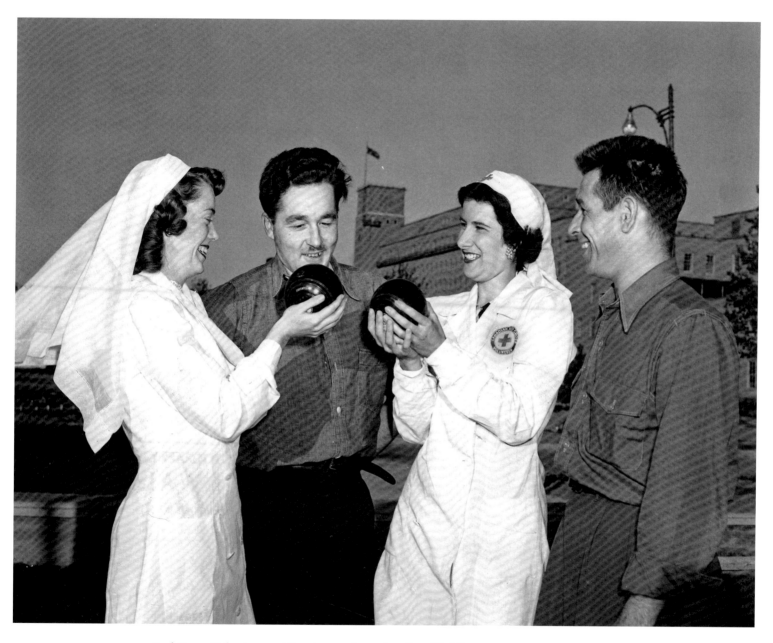

Red Cross Volunteers with veterans, lawn bowling (1950).

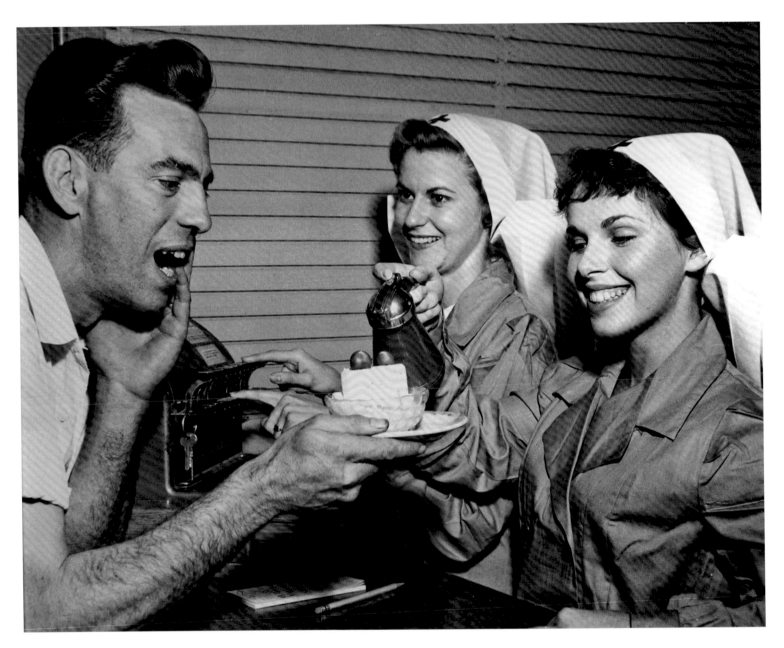

Red Cross volunteers with a veteran.

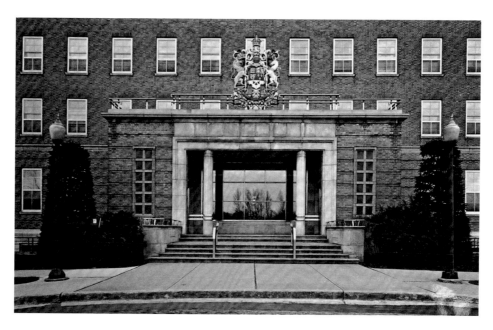

Main Entrance and Royal Coat of Arms of Canada.

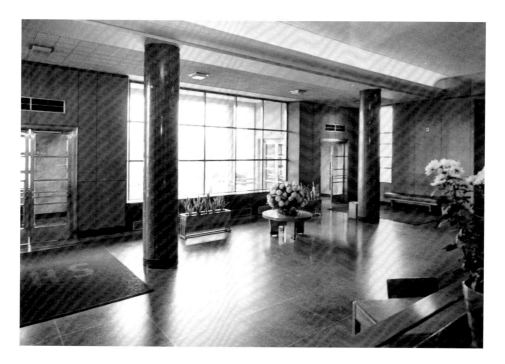

Sunnybrook main lobby, C-Wing (1949).

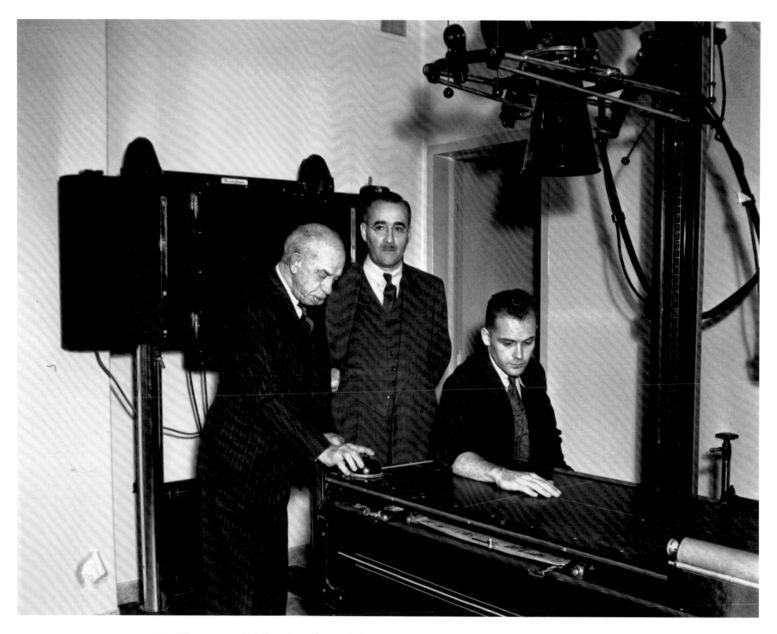

Dr. Thomas and Colonel Hollis with first X-ray machine at Sunnybrook (1948).

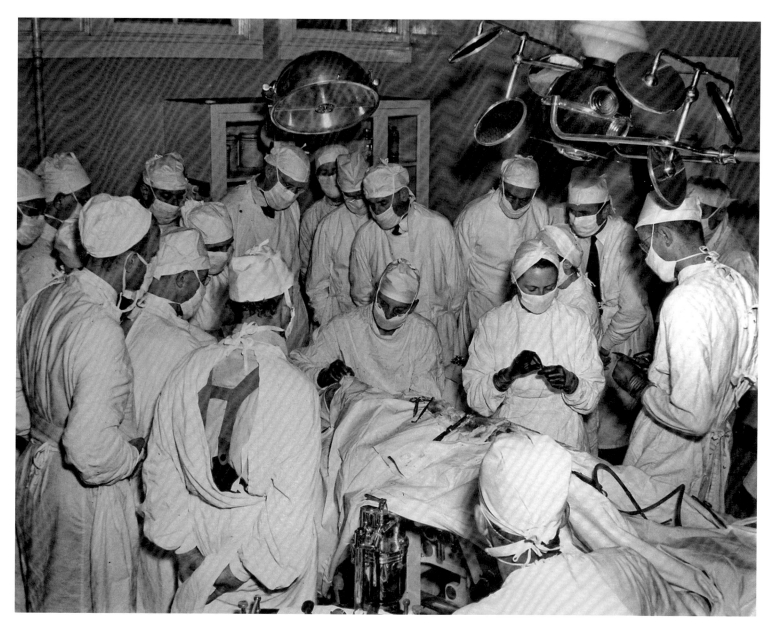

Operating room with numerous learners observing (c. 1950).

Sunnybrook's role as an educational institution began very early in its history. Under the leadership of Dr. Ian Macdonald, a distinguished number of future leaders in medicine from across the country completed part of their postgraduate education at Sunnybrook. Resident education for the University of Toronto was particularly sought after because of the wide spectrum of complex patients and the superb teaching provided by Sunnybrook's medical specialists, most of whom were based at the downtown university teaching hospitals. Despite their part-time status, they created a culture of excellence in patient care and education. They included Dr. David McKenzie (St. Michael's Hospital), Drs. Charlie Brown and Cam Gray (Toronto General Hospital), Dr. Bruce Charles (Toronto East General Hospital), and Dr. Bernie Liebel (Mt. Sinai Hospital). Dr. Arthur Squires (Toronto General Hospital and The Wellesley Hospital), one of Ontario's first haematologists, provided the seminal training for Dr. John Senn, who later became head of Haematology at Sunnybrook.

An impressive group of residents and fellows benefited from the teachers and the patients at Sunnybrook. They included Drs. John Evans, Robert Volpe, Ted Cross, Alex Little, and Hugh Smythe. Dr. Fraser Mustard's pioneering work on atherosclerosis started at Sunnybrook and was later recognized with the Order of Canada. Dr. Ken Brown ultimately established the hospital's first coronary care unit. Throughout the 1950s and 1960s, Medical Grand Rounds were well-attended by Sunnybrook medical staff and by specialists from as far away as Kingston and Hamilton. Regular distinguished guests included Emeritus Professors Dr. William Boyd (Order of Canada), former University Chair of Pathology, and Dr. Duncan Graham, former Sir John and Lady Eaton Professor of Medicine.

Dr. Joseph MacFarlane was the first Surgeon-in-Chief. Dr. J.D. Mills (General surgery) and Dr. Gordon "Papa" Dale (Orthopaedic surgery) transferred from Christie Street and worked full time at Sunnybrook. The remaining members of the attending surgical staff were part-time, drawn from the Toronto teaching hospitals. They included renowned individuals such as Dr. Bill Bigelow (Cardiovascular surgery), Dr. Harry "the horse" Botterell (Neurosurgery), Dr. George Pennal (Orthopaedics), Drs. Hoyle Campbell and Ross Tilley (Plastic surgery), and Dr. Carl "Bubs" Aberhart (Urology)

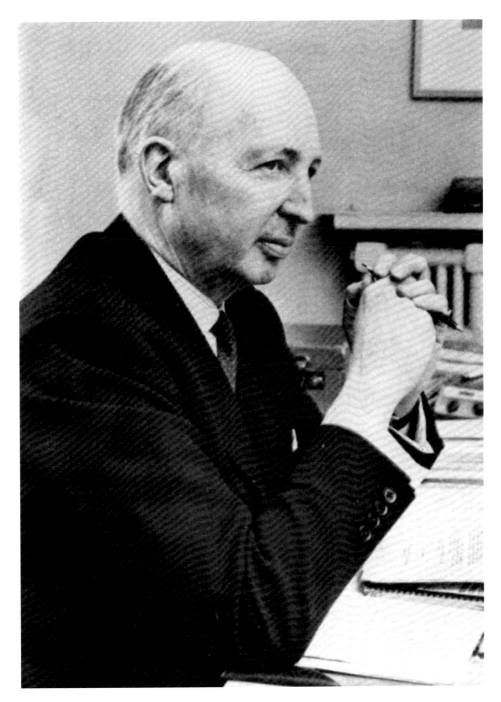

Dr. Ian Macdonald, Sunnybrook's first Physician-in-Chief (1947–66).

who succeeded Dr. MacFarlane as chief. In 1958, Dr. Alan (Al) Harrison joined the full-time staff as the Division Head for General Surgery. He would later become Sunnybrook's third Surgeon-in-Chief.

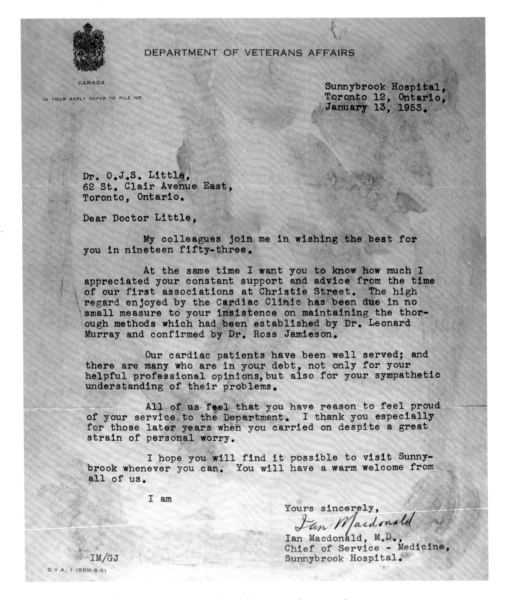

Letter of thanks from Dr. Ian Macdonald to Dr. Oliver Little, 1953.
(Courtesy of Derek Little)

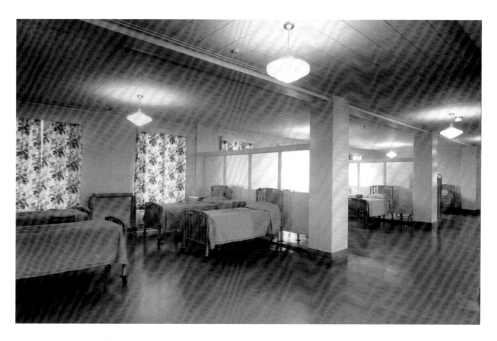

A typical 24-bed ward.

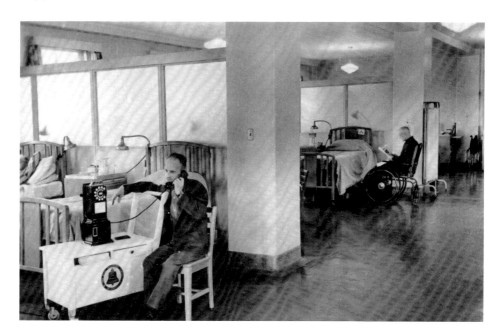

A typical 24-bed ward, with mobile telephone.

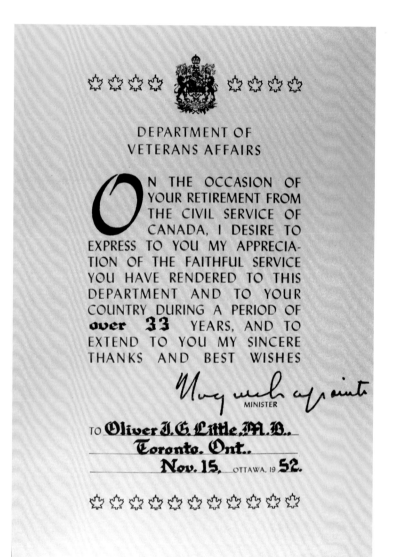

PRAISES SUNNYBROOK

To the Editor of The Star.

Sir: Having been a veteran of the South African War and World War I, I have had occasion to be admitted as a patient into both the old Christie Street hospital and the new Sunnybrook hospital. While convalescing in these hospitals the staff have always been very pleasant and co-operative. I wish to pay tribute to Dr. Little and others who, even beyond the call of duty, minister daily to the needs of veterans who are handicapped through serving their country. The new Sunnybrook hospital seems to have all the finest facilities and accommodation to be desired and certainly is a credit to the country.

RALPH NAYLOR
Oshawa, Ont.

DEPARTMENT OF VETERANS AFFAIRS

ON THE OCCASION OF YOUR RETIREMENT FROM THE CIVIL SERVICE OF CANADA, I DESIRE TO EXPRESS TO YOU MY APPRECIATION OF THE FAITHFUL SERVICE YOU HAVE RENDERED TO THIS DEPARTMENT AND TO YOUR COUNTRY DURING A PERIOD OF **over 33** YEARS, AND TO EXTEND TO YOU MY SINCERE THANKS AND BEST WISHES

MINISTER

TO Oliver J.G. Little, M.B.
Toronto. Ont..
Nov. 15. OTTAWA, 19 52.

LEFT: *Letter to the editor from a Boer War and First World War veteran.*
(Courtesy of Derek Little)

RIGHT: *Certificate of appreciation to Dr. Oliver Little, upon his retirement in 1952.*
(Courtesy of Derek Little)

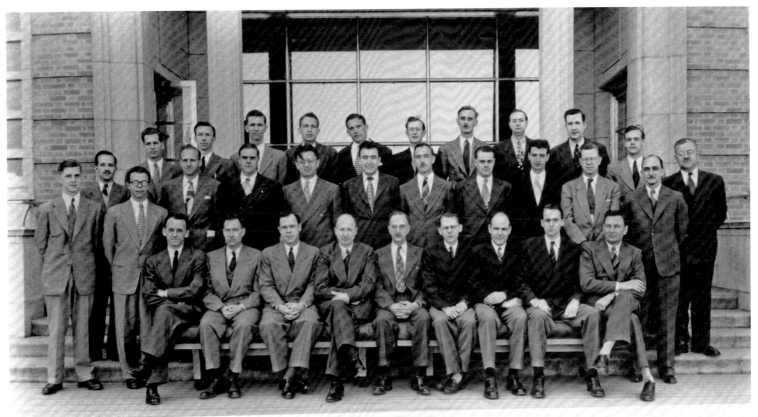

Sunnybrook Hospital
Medical House Staff, 1948-49

Back row: S.G. Strickland, W.E. Boothroyd, J.N. Eydt, D.B. Campbell, O. Kofman, H. Tonning, G.W. Smith, T.E. Hunt, N.H. Rumball, K.P. Turner.

Centre row: J. Rousseau, J.E. Todd, A.M. Park, J. Chmara, A. Sharp, W.A. Young, R.J. Delaney, W.C. Burchill, G.W. Fitzgerald, R.B. Gibb, E.C. Evans.

Front row: D.M. Finlayson, C.G. Cameron, J. Greenblatt, J.D. Armstrong, J.C. Douglas, R.I. Macdonald, Director, K.E. Hollis Superintendent, W.B. Arnup, Resident, J.S. Crawford, H.J. Barnett, J.N. Cunningham.

Medical House Staff, 1948–49, including physicians-in-training.

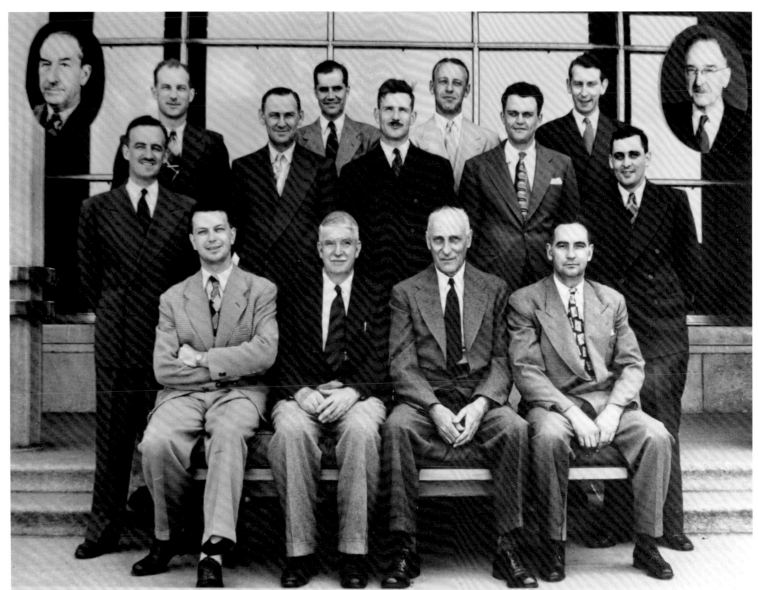

FIRST SURGICAL HOUSE STAFF – SUNNYBROOK HOSPITAL

JUNE 1949

Front Row – S. KLING, G. DALE,(Chief-Orthops) J. D. MILLS, (Chief Gen Surg'y) C. ROBSON
Middle Row – A. JOLICOEUR, F. MacMILLAN, R. CROOME, H. PEARSALL, J. McIVOR.
Rear Row – H. GIBSON, B. WELLS, L. DAVIES, J. AYLWIN.
L. Inset – DR. J.A. MacFARLANE, Director of Surgical Services.
R. Inset – DR. K. E. HOLLIS, Hospital Superintendent.
Absent – R. LOFTHOUSE, W. WALLACE.

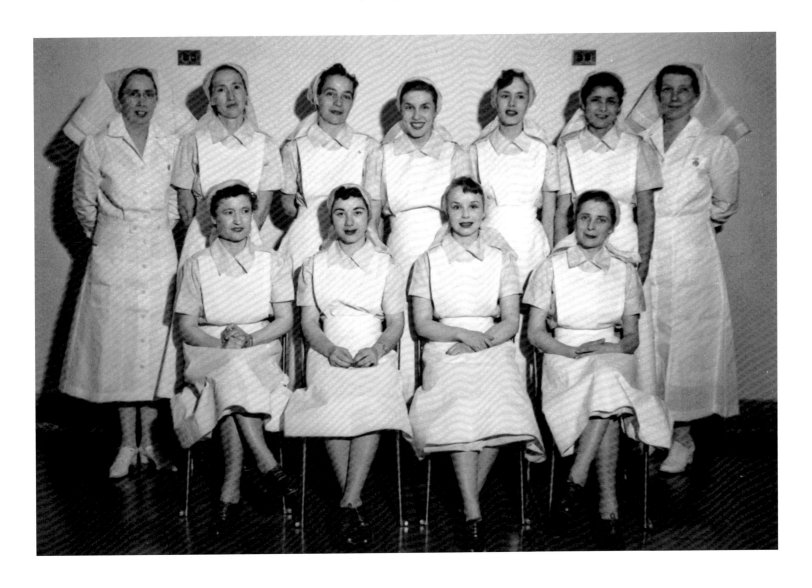

FACING: *First Surgical House Staff, June 1949, including surgeons-in-training.*

ABOVE: *First graduating class of Sunnybrook nursing students receiving their caps, 1952.*

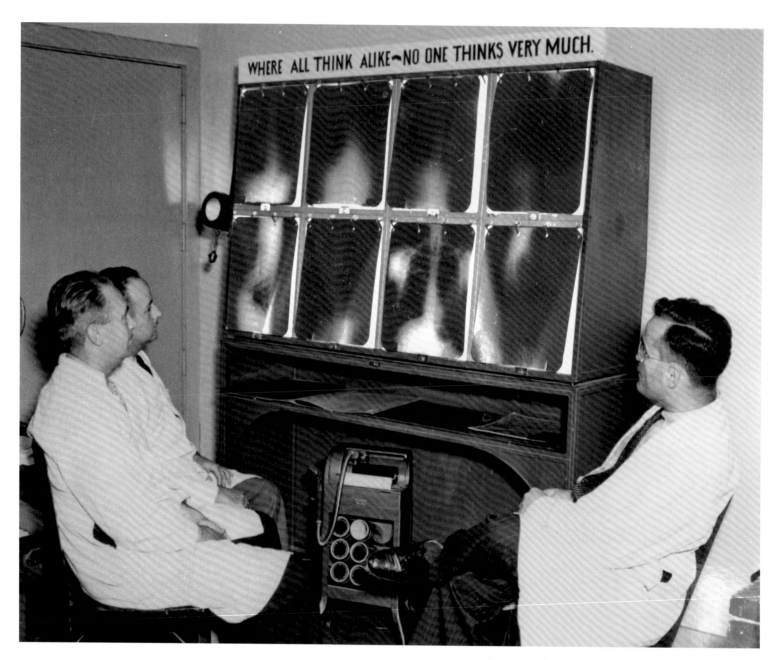

Physicians reviewing X-rays (c. 1960).

Sunnybrook also played a significant role in Otolaryngology in this era. Dr. Cecil Rae, the first department chief, was succeeded in 1966 by Dr. Percy Ireland, who had just retired as the first University of Toronto Professor of Otolaryngology. Dr. Ireland, who had started the Otolaryngology residency training program, assumed the leadership at Sunnybrook for three years to assist it through the transition to a fully affiliated University of Toronto teaching hospital.

Dr. Dan Campbell was the first Chief of Anaesthesia. Several anaesthetists transferred from Christie Street to Sunnybrook. Trainees were typically from the Armed Forces Medical Corps. The second Chief, Dr. Jim Shapley, was a key leader, along with Dr. Al Harrison and nursing leaders, in establishing the first Surgical Intensive Care Unit at Sunnybrook in 1959.

The first Chief of the Department of Neuropsychiatry was Dr. Fred VanNostrand, who had been on staff at Christie Street from 1929–39 before going into the Army Medical Corps. Many veterans were afflicted with "shell shock," which is now known as post-traumatic stress disorder. This disorder became an area of expertise at Sunnybrook.

Dr. Desmond Burke was the first Chief of Radiology. Sunnybrook's department was heavily involved in teaching radiology and benefited from the highest radiology volume in Canada. By 1957 Dr. Burke was succeeded by Dr. Kenneth Hodge.

Nurses have always been an important source of assistance and support in the delivery of medical care at Sunnybrook. The first Director of Nursing, Matron Frances Charlton, was instrumental in ensuring that nurses were vital members of the health care team. Under her guidance, the Nursing Assistant Program provided a generation of nurses with education at Sunnybrook.

Doris Kent became the second Director of Nursing and for many years played a key role in ensuring the continued high standards of care provided by the nursing staff.

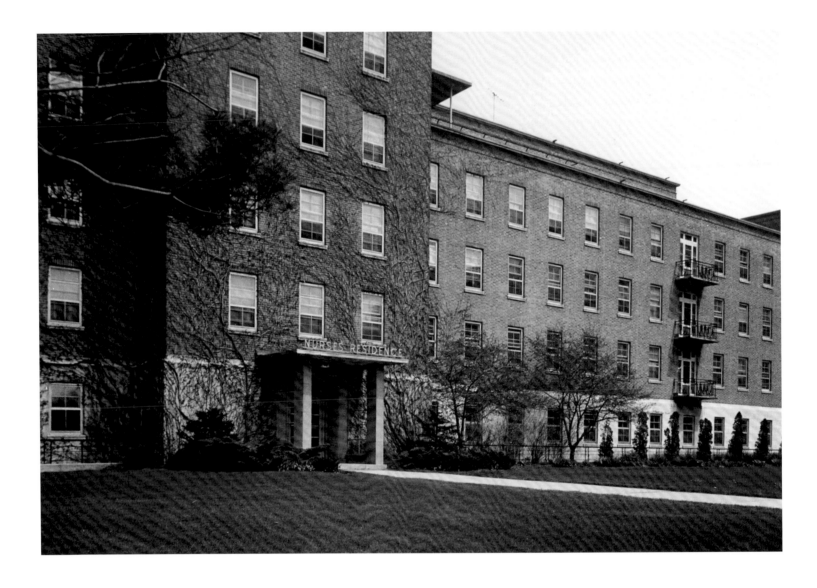

ABOVE: *Nurses' residence, currently H-wing.*

FACING: *Doris Kent, Director of Nursing.*

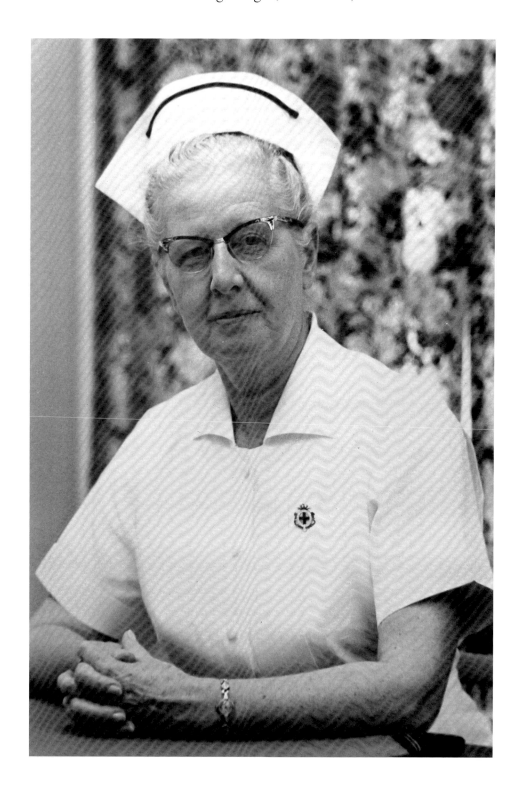

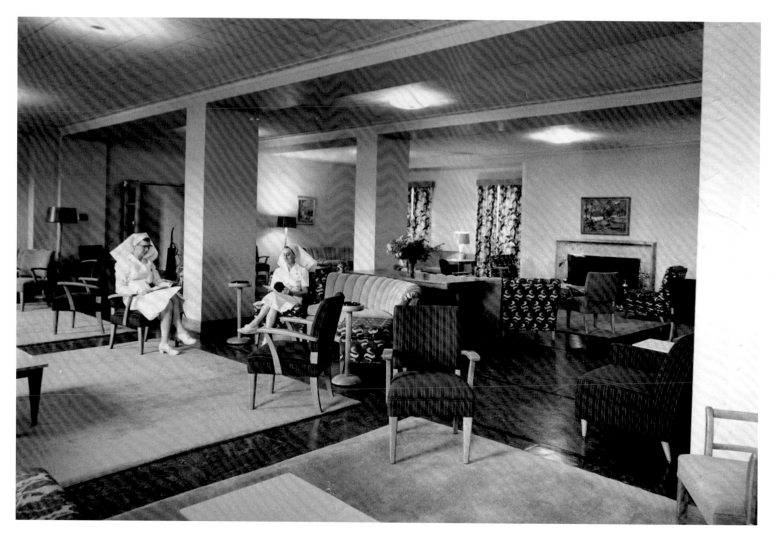

Nurses' lounge.

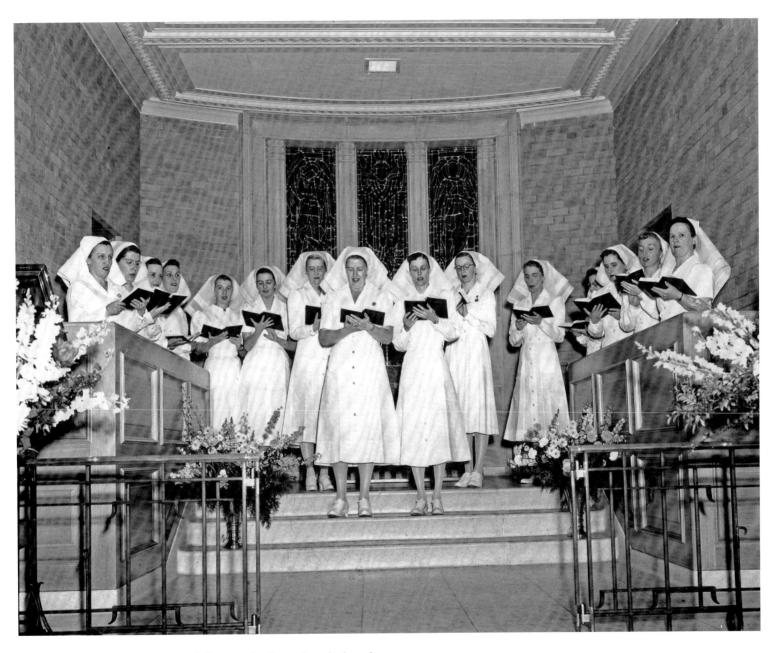

Nurses' choir at the Sunnybrook chapel.

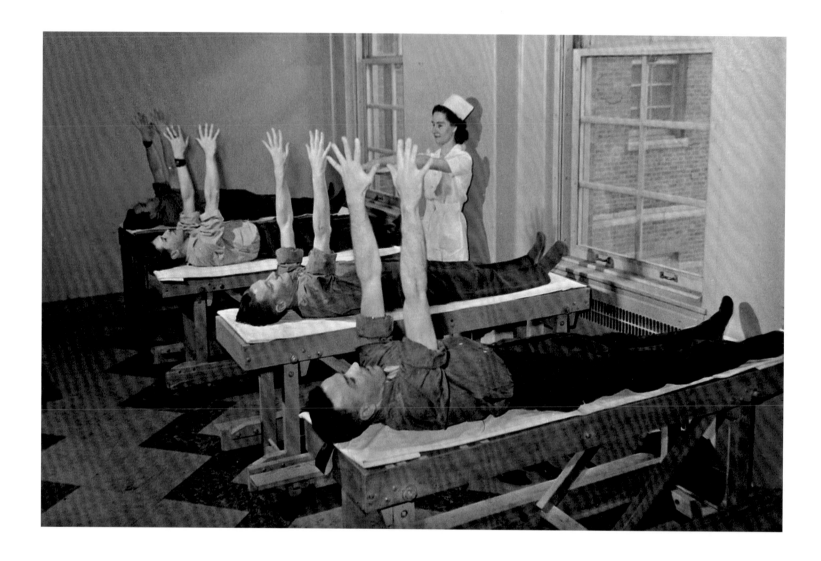

ABOVE: *Nurse with veterans during physiotherapy exercises.*

FACING: *Miss Freethy with Mr. Wambolt on the physiotherapy treadmill (1952).*

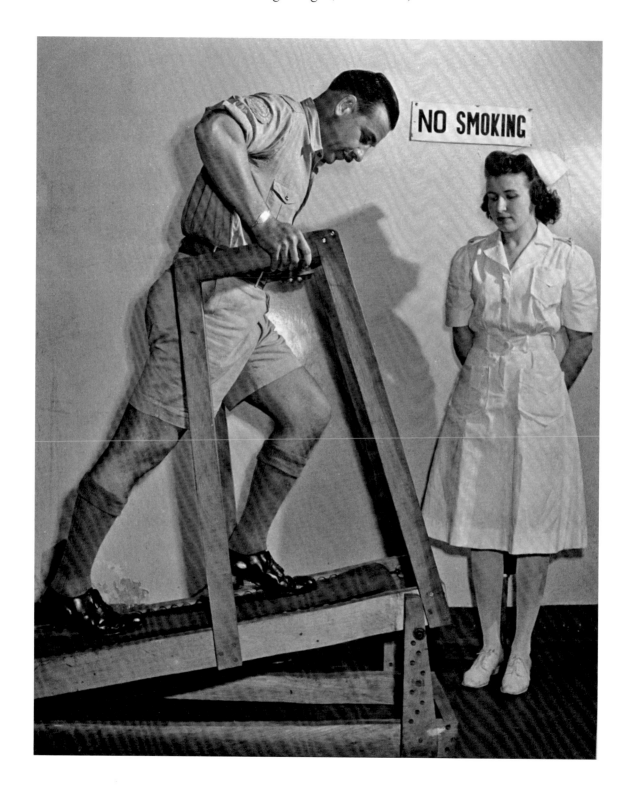

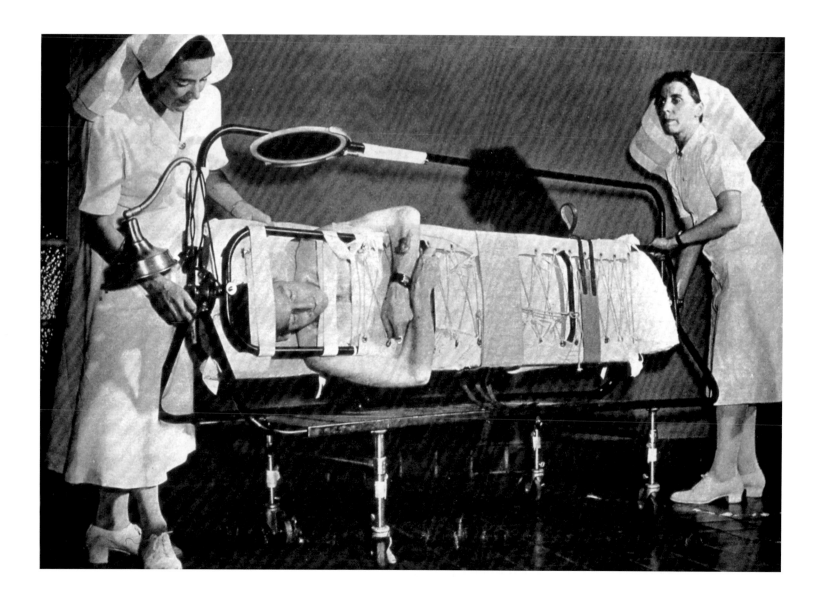

ABOVE: *Nurses Vanderwell and Lethbridge rotating a veteran with a Stryker frame.*

FACING: *Nurses with veteran in the therapy bath.*

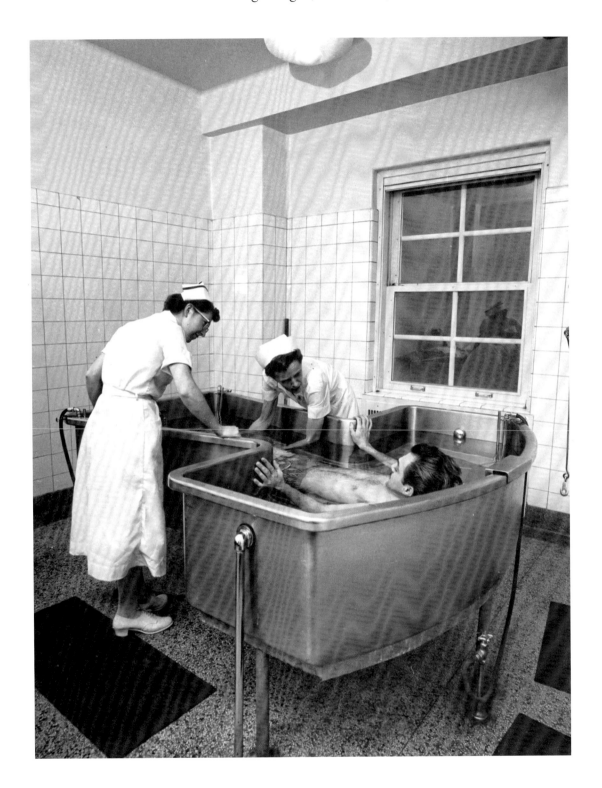

In 1953, Dr. Clement McLeod was appointed as the second Hospital Superintendent. He supervised the creation of the first Clinical Investigation Unit. By 1954, 25 research projects were underway in the facility.

The clinical care at Sunnybrook was originally focused on meeting the needs of the veterans. The veteran population provided some unique opportunities for Sunnybrook surgeons, who developed a national reputation for reconstructive surgical procedures for severe burns and musculoskeletal injuries, including amputations.

An outstanding group of faculty with expertise in rheumatic diseases and arthritis was led by Drs. Wallace Graham, Almon Fletcher, Don Graham, and Metro Ogryzlo. In 1962, this led to the creation at Sunnybrook of Canada's first Rheumatic Diseases Unit. Later in the decade, this unit relocated to The Wellesley Hospital and drew upon former Sunnybrook fellows such as Dr. Hugh Smythe as future leaders.

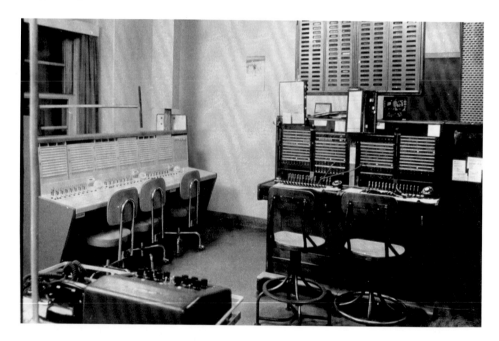

ABOVE: *Main hospital switchboard.*

FACING: *Clinic room (c. 1950).*

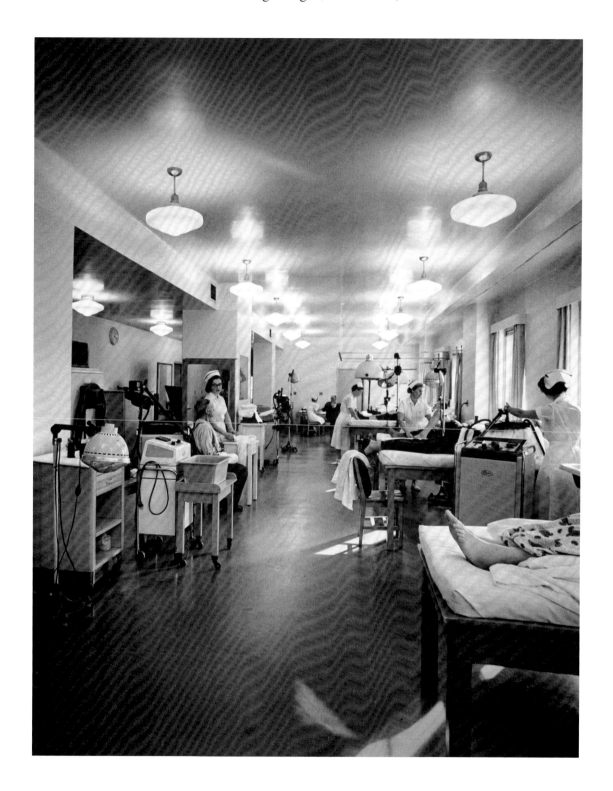

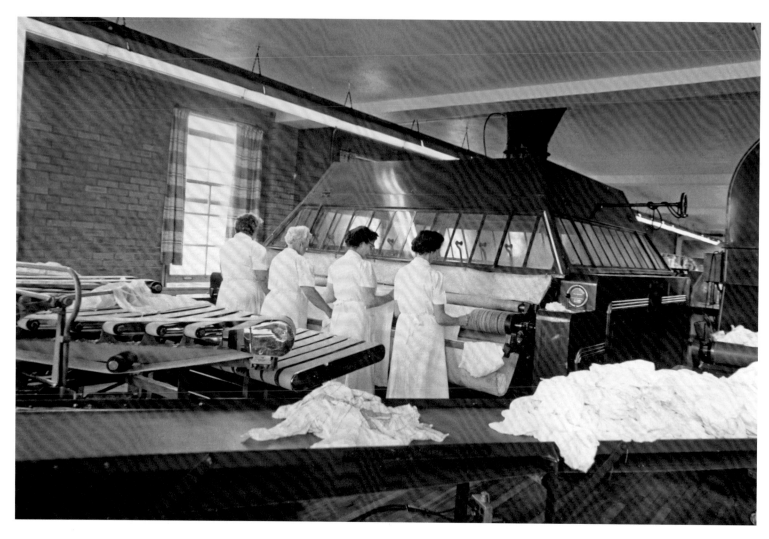

Laundry facilities.

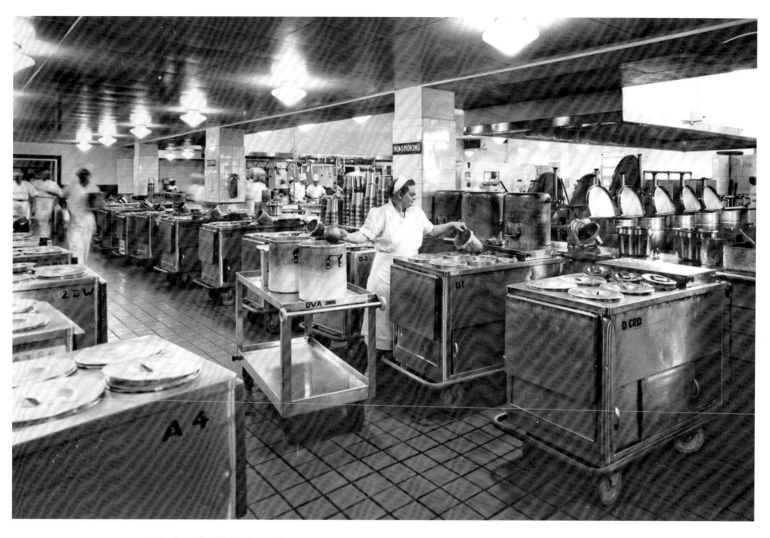

Kitchen facilities (1949).

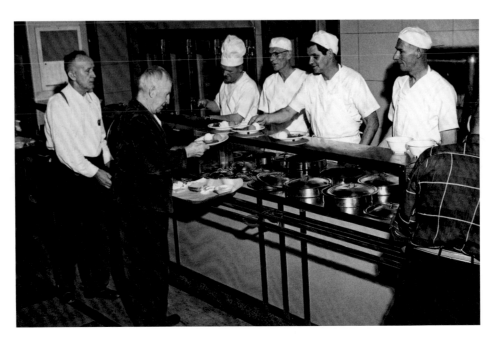

At the counter in the Veterans' Canteen (c. 1950).

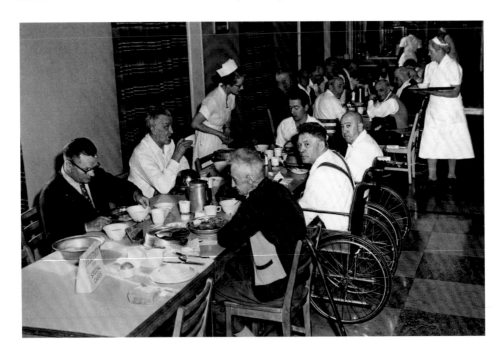

Dining Hall (1949).

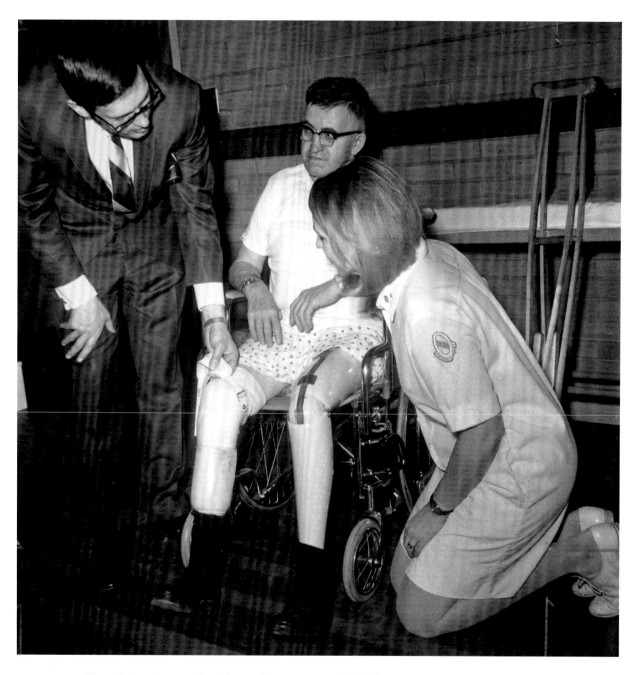

Examining the prosthetic legs of a veteran with double amputation.

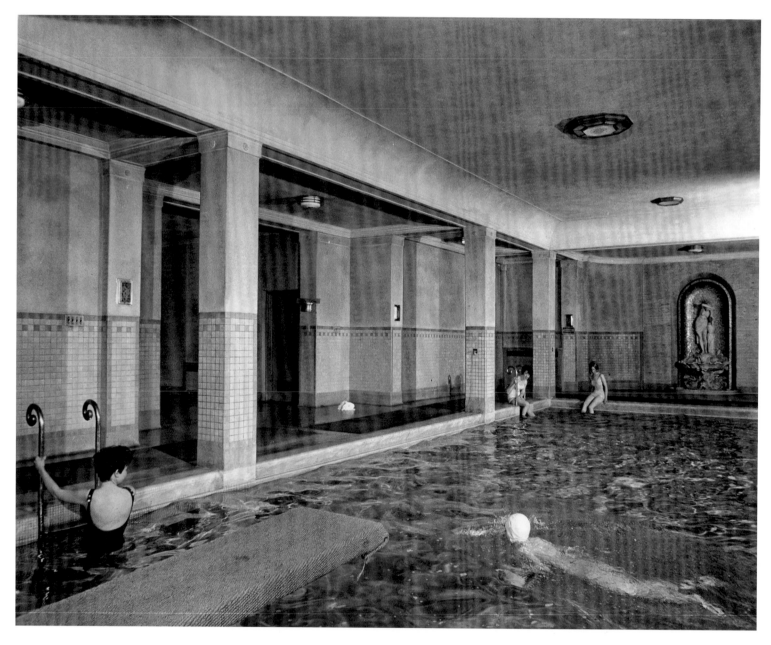

Swimming pool at the Divadale Estate (1955).

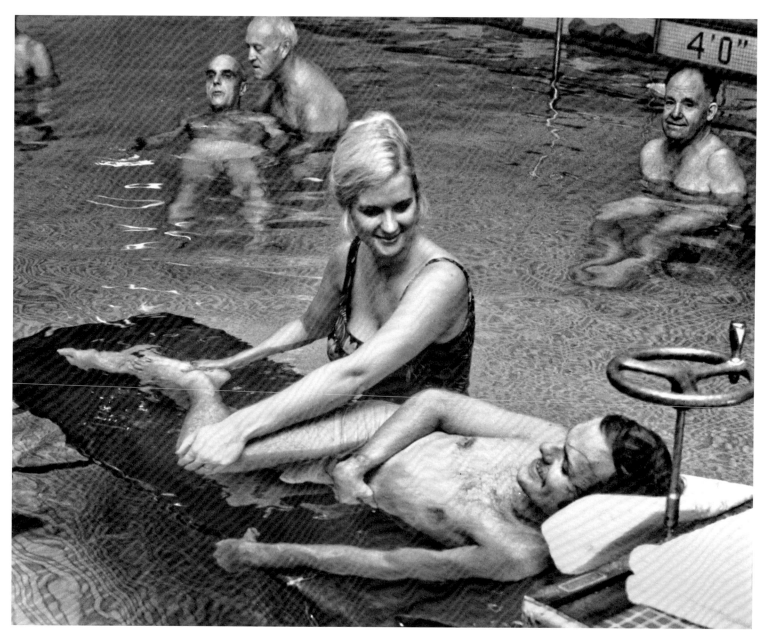

Physiotherapy at the therapy pool.

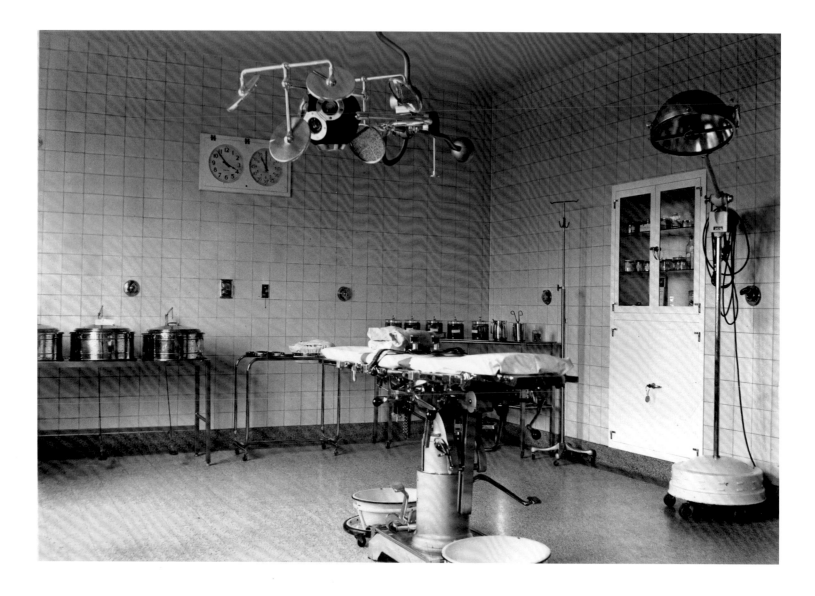

Above: *Operating room (c. 1950).*

Facing: *Dr. J.M. Shapley, Chief of Anaesthesia (1955–68).*

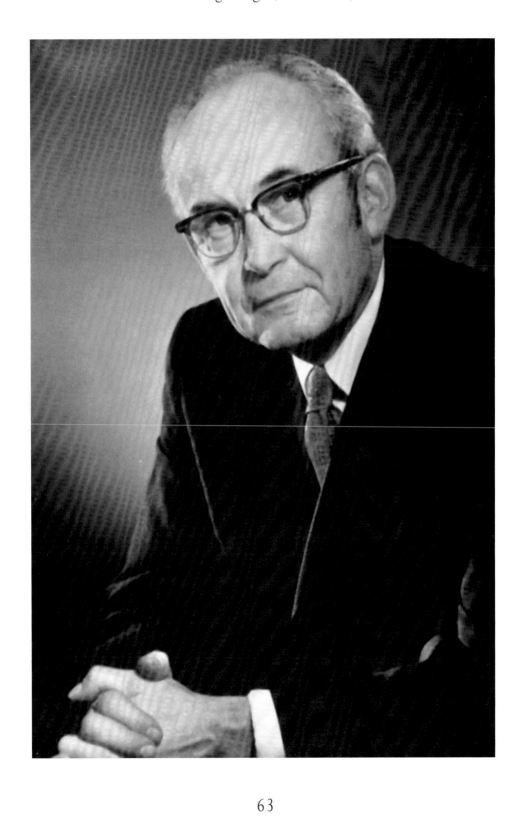

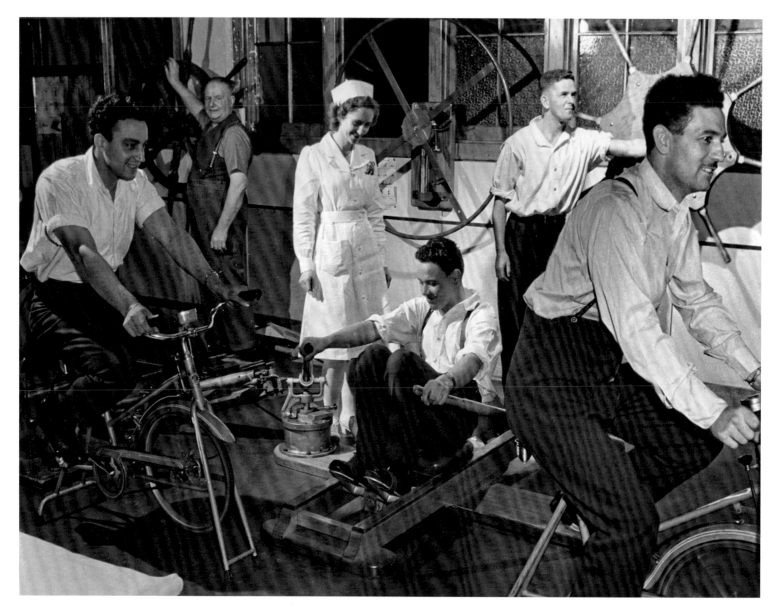

Veterans on various physiotherapy devices.

Many veterans benefited from the services of the Physical Medicine Unit and the Paraplegia Unit. This unit was a combined effort of Drs. Botterell and Aberhart from Surgery and Drs. Al Jousse and William Geisler from Rehabilitation Medicine. The unit also provided learning opportunities for trainees in physical therapy and occupational therapy. The Prosthetics Unit was known nationwide for the design and manufacture of artificial limbs, skull plates, ears, eyes, noses, and other appliances required for disabled veterans.

In 1954, Sunnybrook demographics showed that it had 9,912 in-patients with a total of 444,401 patient days. In the outpatient clinics, 64,287 patients were seen, an average of 233 visits per day. Attending physicians and surgeons numbered 130. There were 18 research staff members.

During that era, the veterans were honoured by the visits of many dignitaries and celebrities. In 1951, HRH Princess Elizabeth visited Sunnybrook, and eight years later she paid a return visit as Her Majesty Queen Elizabeth II. In 1956, Governor General Vincent Massey was a welcomed visitor. Celebrity visitors of that era included Dame Vera Lynn, Bob Hope, Jimmy Durante, Roy Rogers, and Red Skelton.

By the early 1960s, with occupancy rates diminishing and almost half of the treatment beds occupied by chronic-care patients, the federal government began to reconsider its role in the operation of Canada's veterans' hospitals. A plan was devised to transfer the veterans' facilities to universities with medical schools. This would also help to alleviate community hospital bed shortages.

On October 1, 1966, the Government of Canada transferred Sunnybrook to the University of Toronto for one silver dollar, beginning Sunnybrook's official affiliation with the University of Toronto. Legislation created the Sunnybrook Hospital Act, which was the culmination of many years of behind-the-scenes activity. Key individuals in the formation of the act included Professor Sidney Smith, former President of the University of Toronto; Henry Borden, Chair of the Board of Governors, University of Toronto; Dr. John Hamilton, Dean of the Faculty of Medicine; the Honourable Roger Teillet, Minister of Veterans Affairs; Budd H. Rieger, the hospital's first Chair of the

Board; Dr. John Evans, University of Toronto, who drafted the mission statement; and the Honourable John Robarts, Premier of Ontario. Norman Bell, a relative of Alice Kilgour, was instrumental in obtaining the permission of the Kilgour heirs for the transfer. He became one of the founding board members and ultimately became Chair of the Board in 1972. Dr. J.K. Morrison, who had been Superintendent since 1962, was appointed as the hospital's first Executive Director.

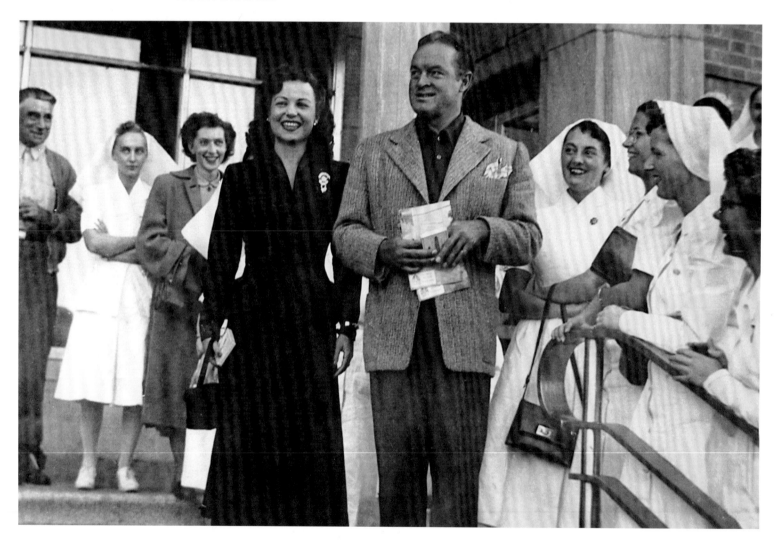

Bob Hope visits Sunnybrook (1948).

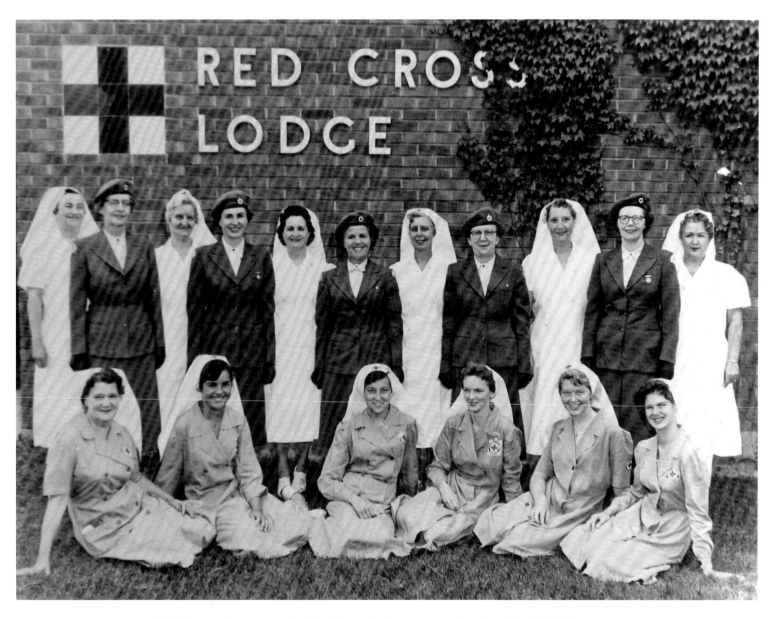

Red Cross volunteers at the Red Cross Lodge preparing for the visit of HRH Queen Elizabeth II (1959).

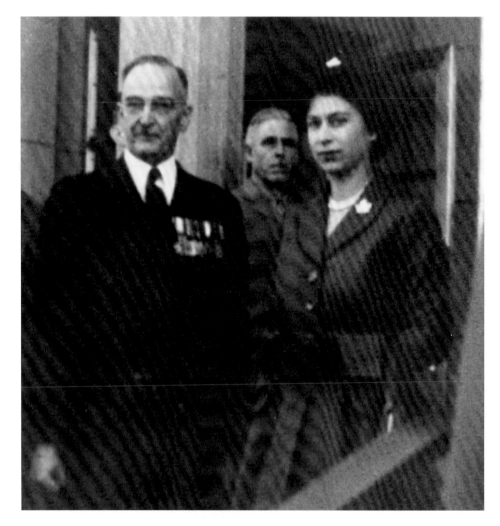

HRH Princess Elizabeth with Colonel Karl Hollis, Sunnybrook Superintendent (1951).

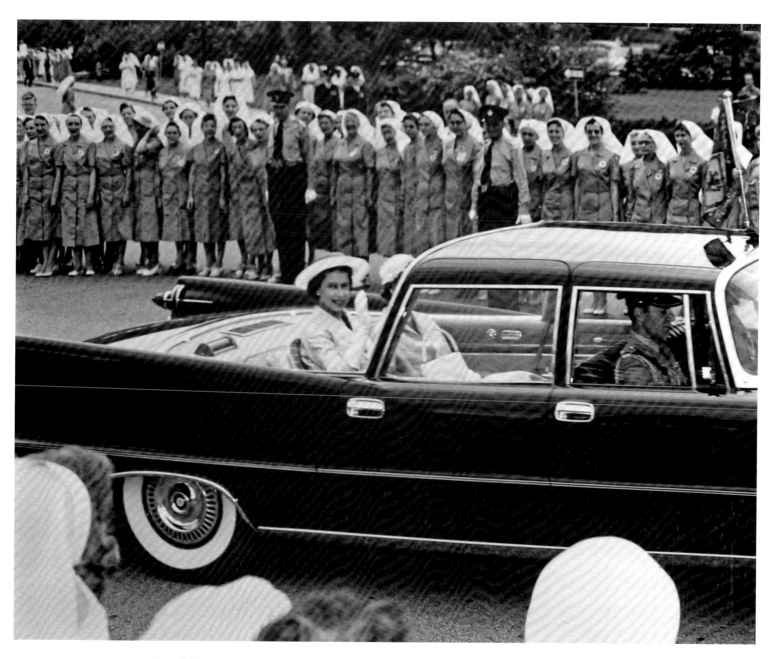

Royal Visit, 1959 — HRH Queen Elizabeth II with Red Cross volunteers in background.

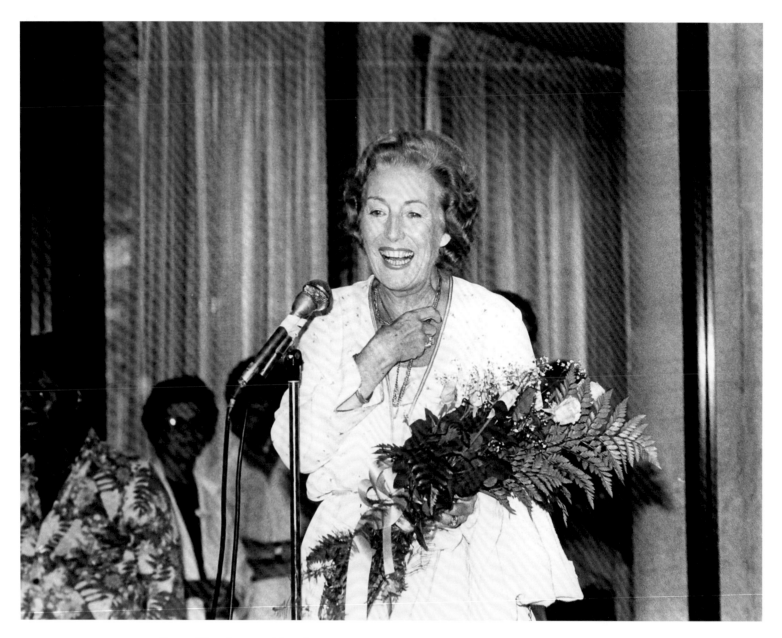

Dame Vera Lynn visiting the veterans.

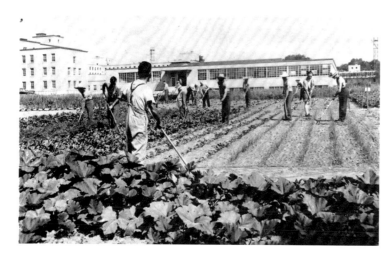

LEFT: *Tending to the patients' garden (1949).*

BELOW: *Veterans on the sunroof (1949).*

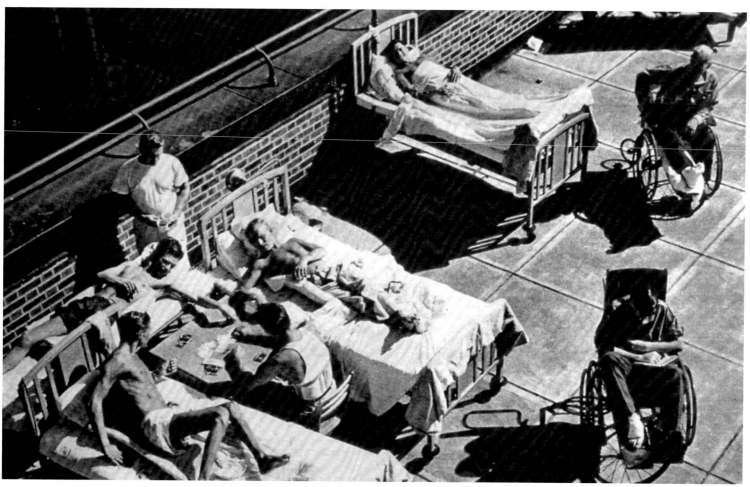

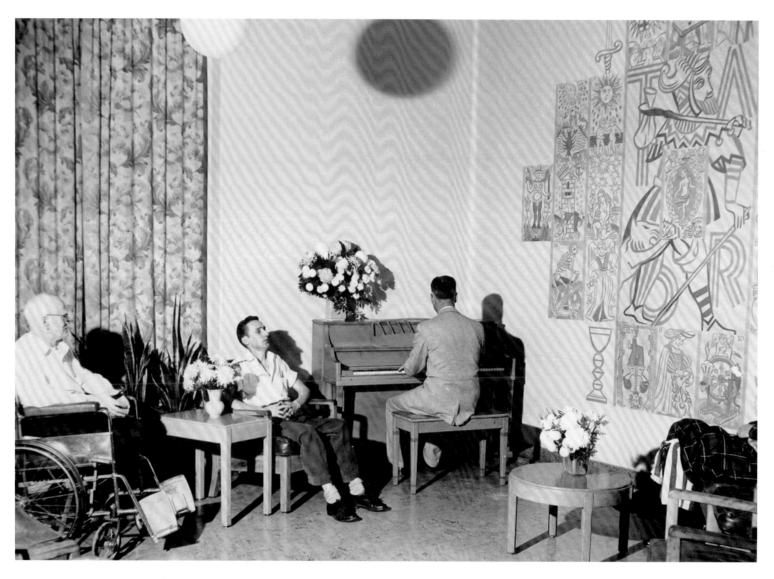

Playing piano in the lounge.

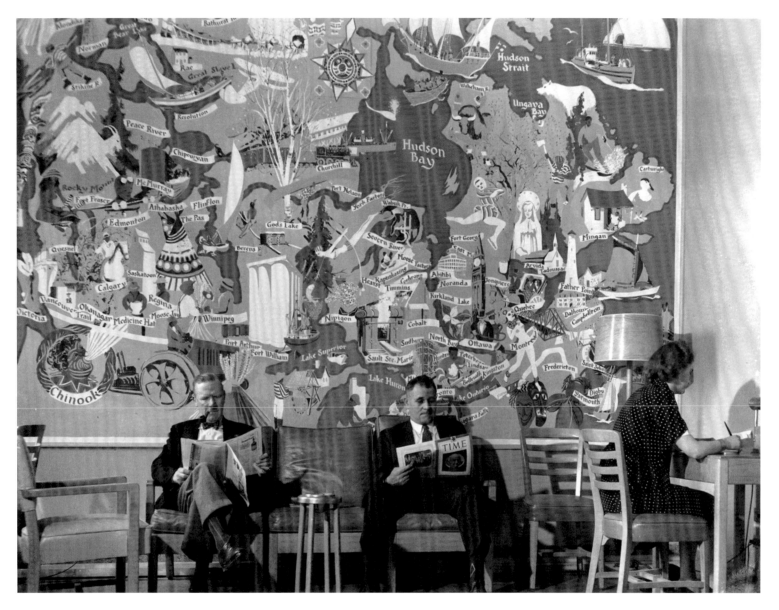

Mural of Canada in the lounge (1949).

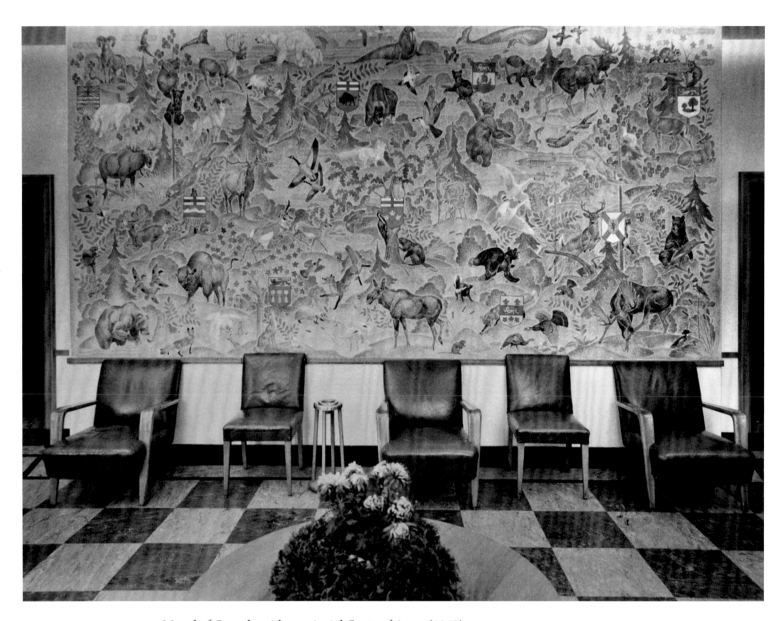

Mural of Canada with provincial Coats of Arms (1949).

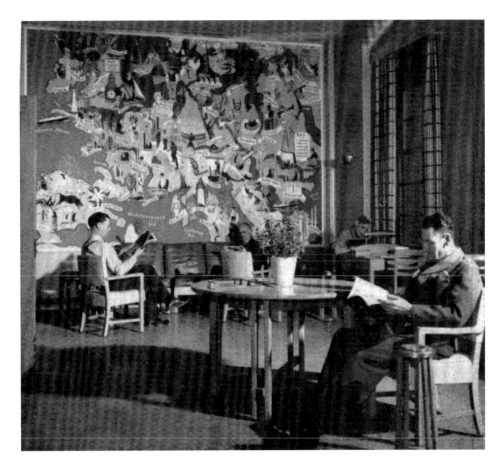

Mural painted by Angus MacDonald.

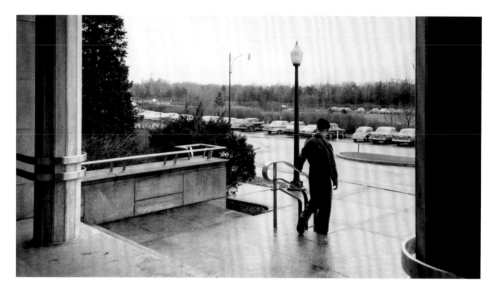

A lone soldier on the main entrance steps (1949).

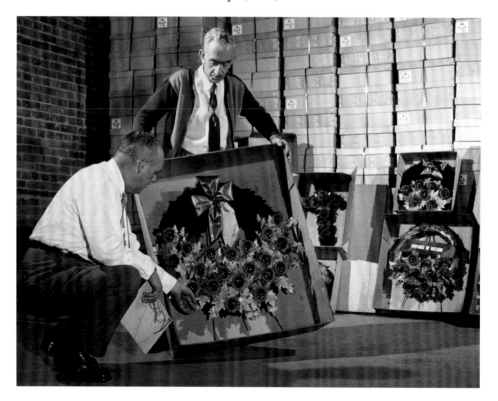

Preparing for Remembrance Day.

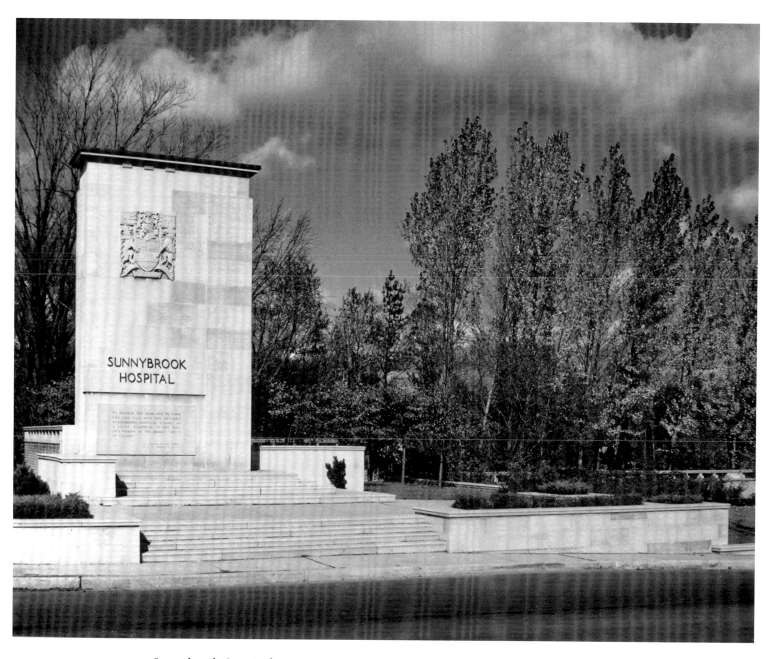

Sunnybrook Cenotaph.

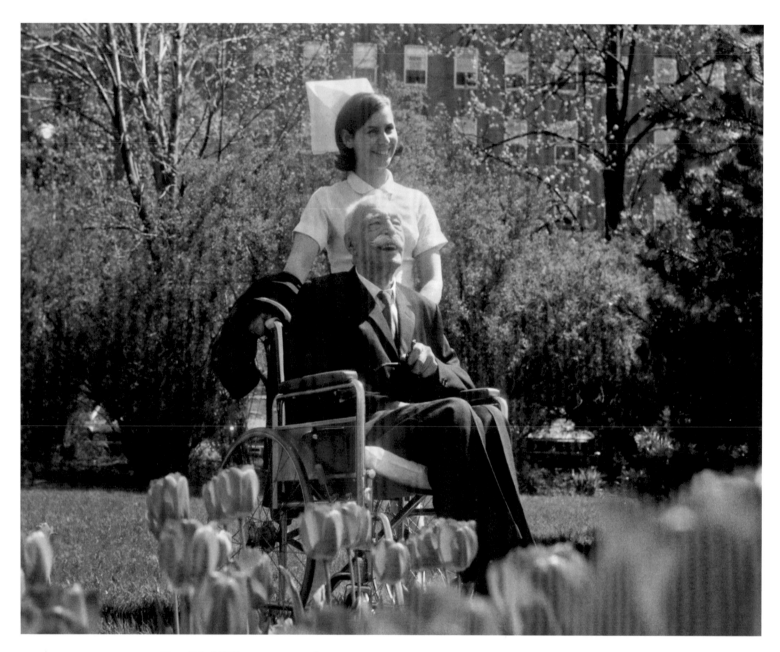

First World War veteran and nurse.

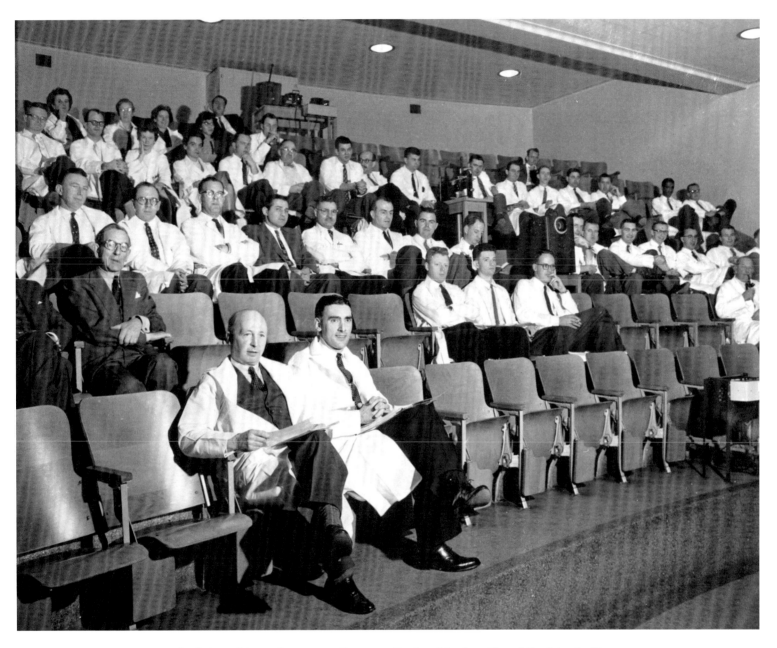

Medical Grand Rounds, c. 1959. First row, Dr. Ian Macdonald and Dr. John Stalker, Chief Medical Resident; Second row, first left, Dr. William Boyd.

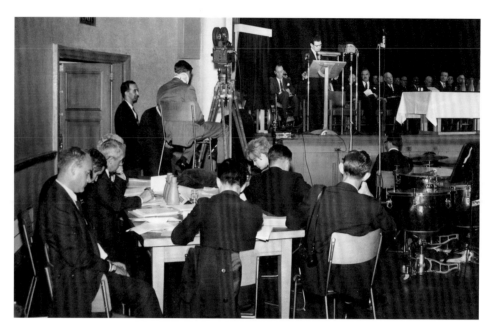

Department of Veterans Affairs transfer of Sunnybrook Hospital to the University of Toronto. Ceremony held in Warriors Hall, October 1, 1966.

The Honourable Roger Teillet, Minister of Veterans Affairs, and Honourable John Robarts, Premier of Ontario, unveiling the dedication plaque at the transfer of Sunnybrook from the Department of Veterans Affairs to the University of Toronto, October 1, 1966.

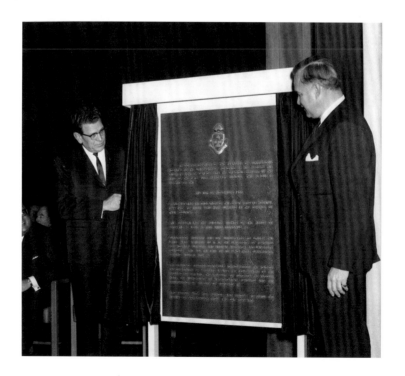

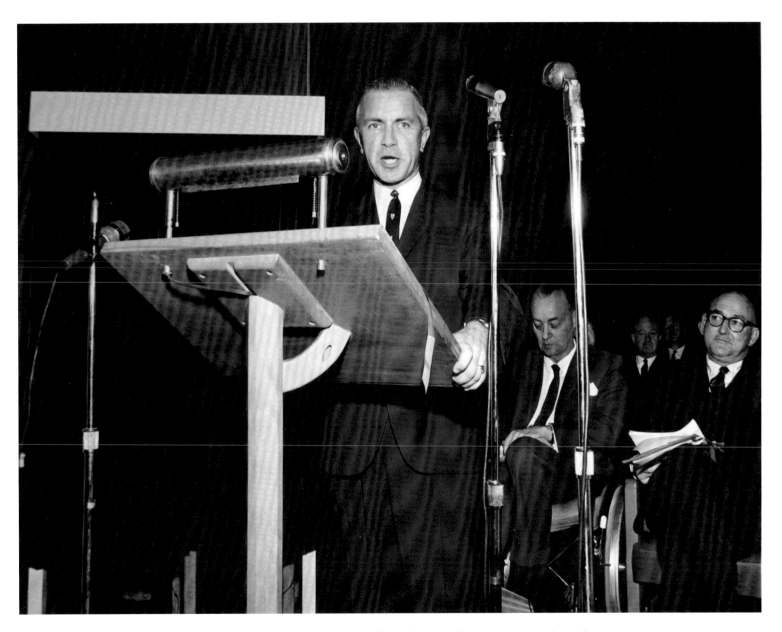

William R. Allen, chair of the Municipality of Metropolitan Toronto at the podium during the transfer ceremony, October 1, 1966.

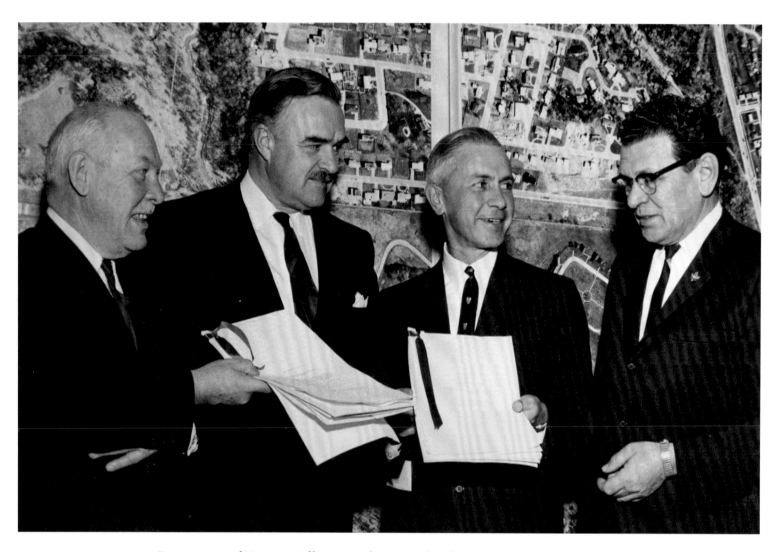

Department of Veterans Affairs transfers Sunnybrook Hospital to the University of Toronto, October 1, 1966. Left to right: Henry Borden, Chair of the University of Toronto Board of Governors; Honourable John Robarts, Premier of the Province of Ontario; Dr. John Sword, University of Toronto Provost; a Honourable Roger Teillet, Minister of Veterans Affairs.

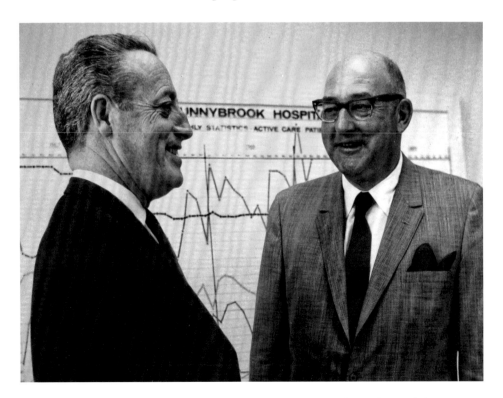

WARRIORS HALL

COMMEMORATING THE ROLE OF SUNNYBROOK AS
A VETERANS HOSPITAL, 1944 - 1966, THIS AUDITORIUM
IS NAMED IN HONOUR OF VETERANS OF THE ARMED FORCES
AND IS DEDICATED ON THIS 25th DAY OF OCTOBER 1966
IN REMEMBRANCE OF THEIR GALLANTRY AND SACRIFICES.

Warriors' Hall dedication plaque, October 25, 1966.

Dr. J.K. Morrison, Superintendent, and Mr. B.H. Rieger, first Chair of the Board of Trustees.

CHAPTER 3

Birth and Growth of a Major Teaching Hospital (1967–1998)

THE MONTHS FOLLOWING THE TRANSITION were a whirlwind of activity. A new Board of Directors had to be formed, new bylaws, policies, and procedures were developed and contracts were signed. Major contributors to this process included Dr. Kemp Morrison, Mr. Bud Dryer, Mr. Norman Bell, and Mr. Aubrey Russell.

The Medical Dental Staff Association was formed. Its first President was Dr. Percy Ireland (Otolaryngology). Other directors of the association included Drs. Alfie Farmer (Surgery), Jim Shapley (Anaesthesia), Jim Sean (Medicine), and Al Harrison (Surgery). Dr. Fred Kergin was the associate dean on site and represented the University of Toronto.

After the appointment of Dr. Al Harrison as Chief of Surgery, the late 1960s witnessed the arrival of several new surgical division leaders, such as Dr. Martin Barkin (Urology), Dr. Marvin Tile (Orthopaedics), Dr. Glen Taylor (General and Thoracic surgery), Dr. Joe Gruss (Plastic surgery), and Dr. Charles Tator (Neurosurgery).

The Physician-in-Chief after the transition was Dr. John Paterson. The key division leaders he recruited made a lasting impact on the hospital. They included Drs. Art Chisholm (Cardiology), John Senn (Haematology), Edgar (Ted) Ritcey (Respirology), Hugh Little (Rheumatology), Carl Saiphoo (Nephrology), Bob Sheppard (Endocrinology), and Carl Wyse (Dermatology), who was soon followed as division head by Dr. Robert (Bob) Lester.

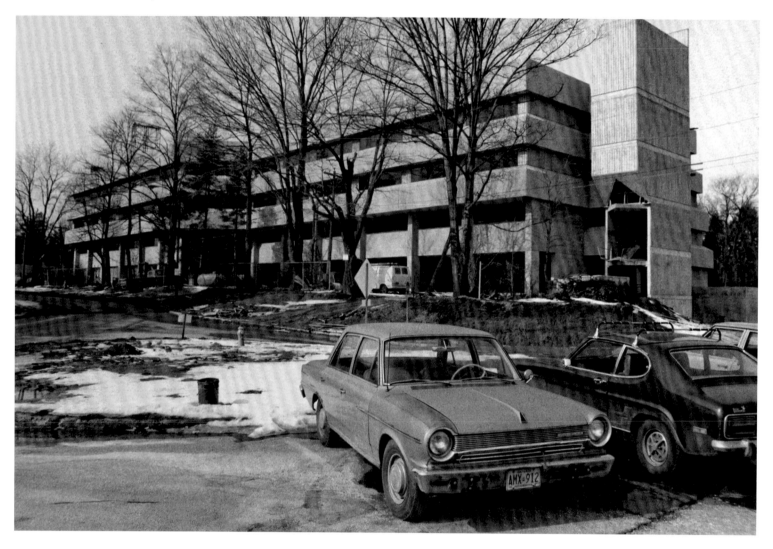

Construction of K-Wing veterans building.

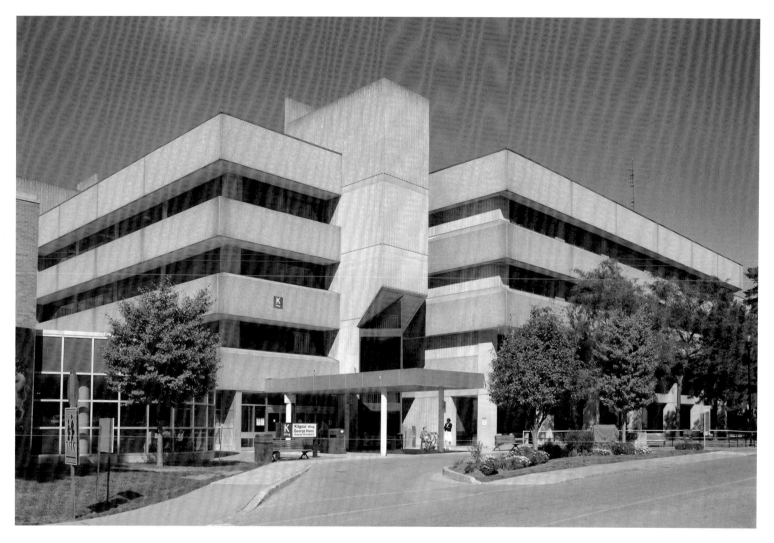

K-Wing (1974).

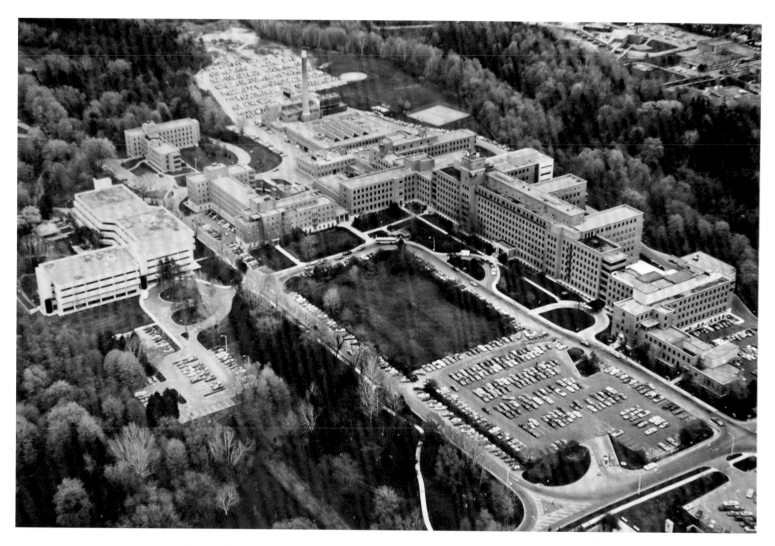

Aerial view of Sunnybrook (1976).

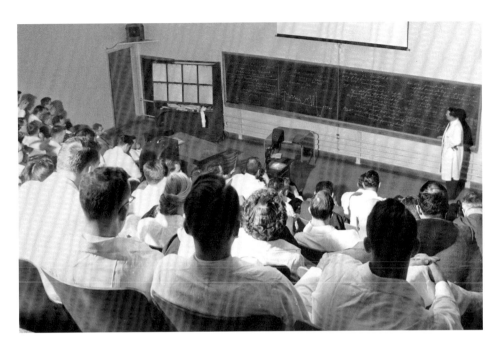

Dr. John Senn, lecturing.

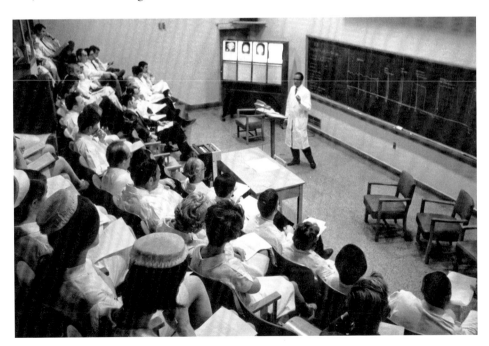

Dr. Carl Saiphoo, lecturing to a multi-professional audience.

The diagnostic departments were led into the new era by a remarkable group of individuals who had a passion for clinical care and teaching. They included Drs. Aaron Malkin (Clinical chemistry), Ian Duncan (Microbiology), Peter Pinkerton (Laboratory haematology), Bruce Cruickshank (Pathology), and Donald McRae (Radiology).

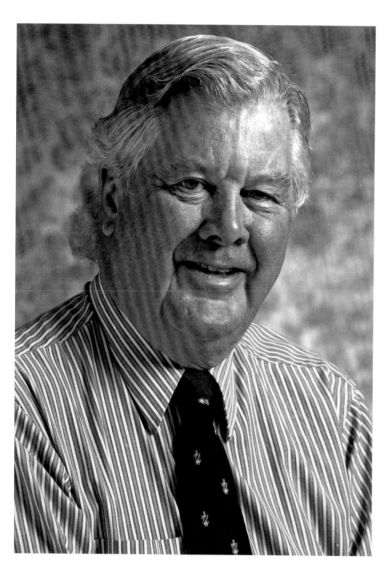

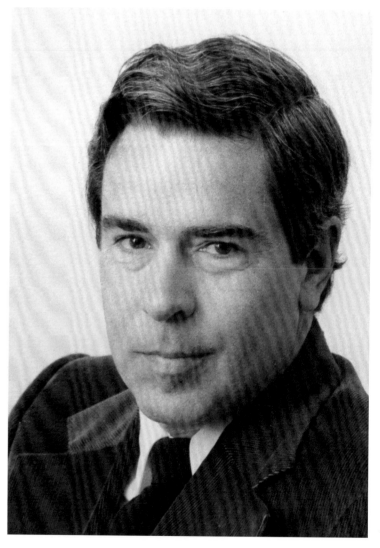

Dr. Peter Pinkerton, Chief of Laboratory Medicine (1967–99).

Dr. Donald Cowan, Chief of Medicine (1974–86).

Dr. Donald McRae, a leading international figure in the radiology of the cervical spine and skull base, was recruited from the Montreal Neurological Institute and McGill University to become Sunnybrook's Chief of Radiology in 1968. He was succeeded by Dr. John Campbell and then Dr. Harry Shulman.

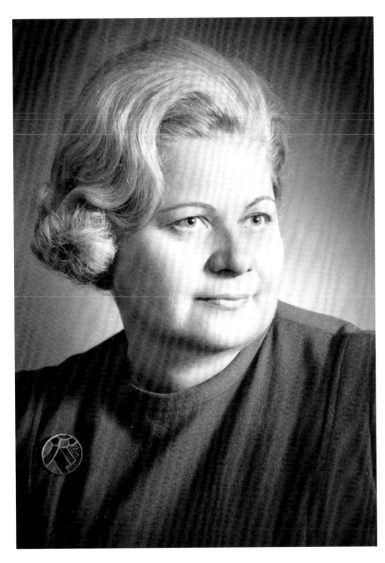

Dorothy Wylie, Director of Nursing (1978–87).

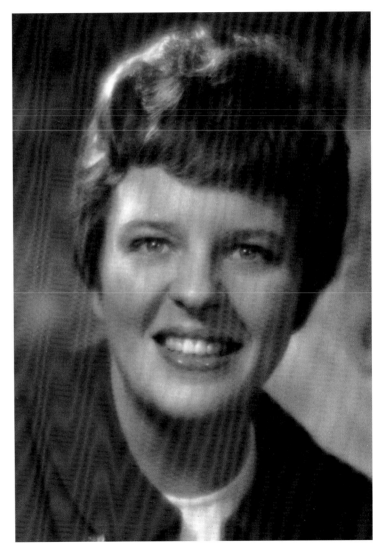

Marian Lorenz, Sunnybrook employee in various areas for over 50 years, starting June 6, 1954.

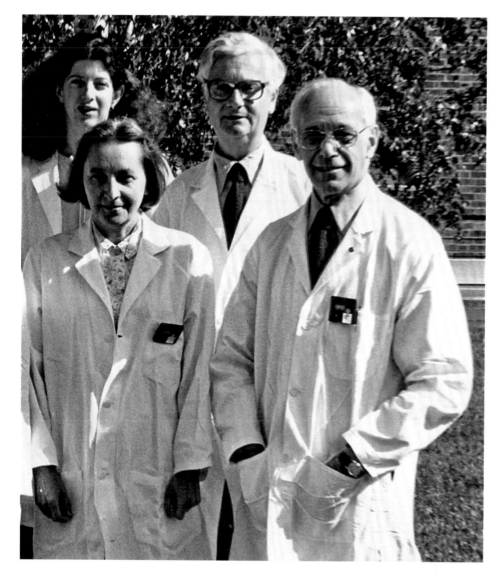

Dr. Dina Malkin and Dr. Aaron Malkin, Chief of Clinical Biochemistry (1962–90).

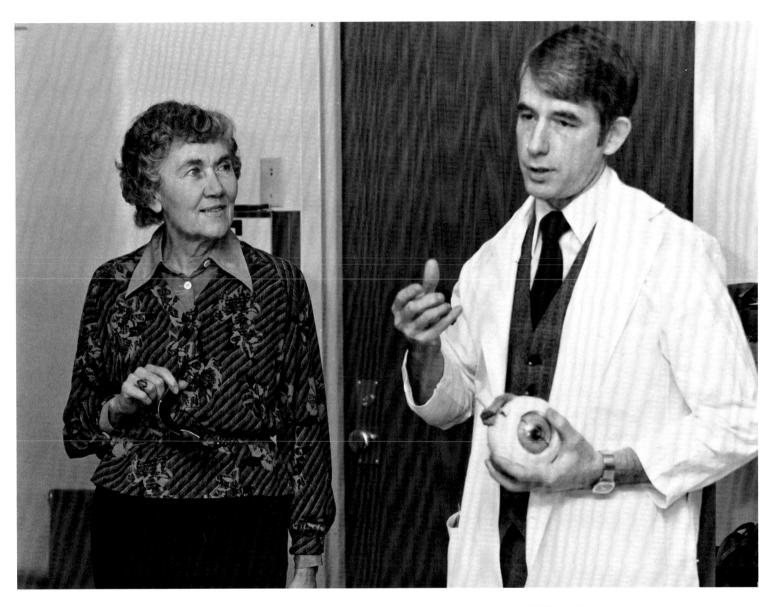

Grateful corneal transplant recipient, Elizabeth Leadbeater and Dr. William Dixon,
Chief of Ophthalmology (1987–2010).

While he was at McGill University, Dr. Edward (Eddie) Kingstone was the first psychiatrist in Canada to use lithium for bipolar disorder. His recruitment to Sunnybrook as Chief of Psychiatry in 1971 was a signal that Sunnybrook's academic reputation was developing rapidly. Dr. Kingstone went on to pioneer Antabuse implants for alcoholism.

Dr. Hugh Barber became the Chief of Otolaryngology in 1969. In addition to establishing a unique dizziness clinic, Dr. Barber also recruited Dr. Julian Nedzelski, who had special expertise in the management of acoustic neuromas and cochlear implants.

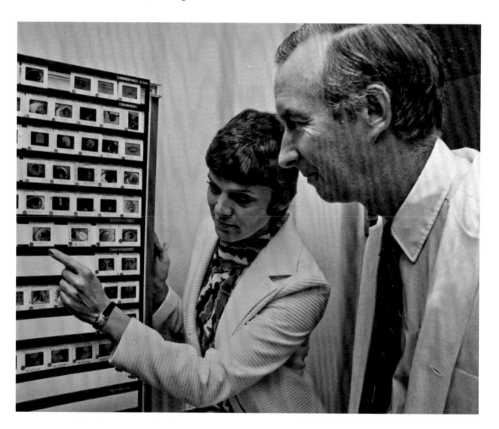

Anne Sloan, Eye Clinic Charge Nurse, and Dr. J.S. Speakman, Chief of Ophthalmology (1969–88).

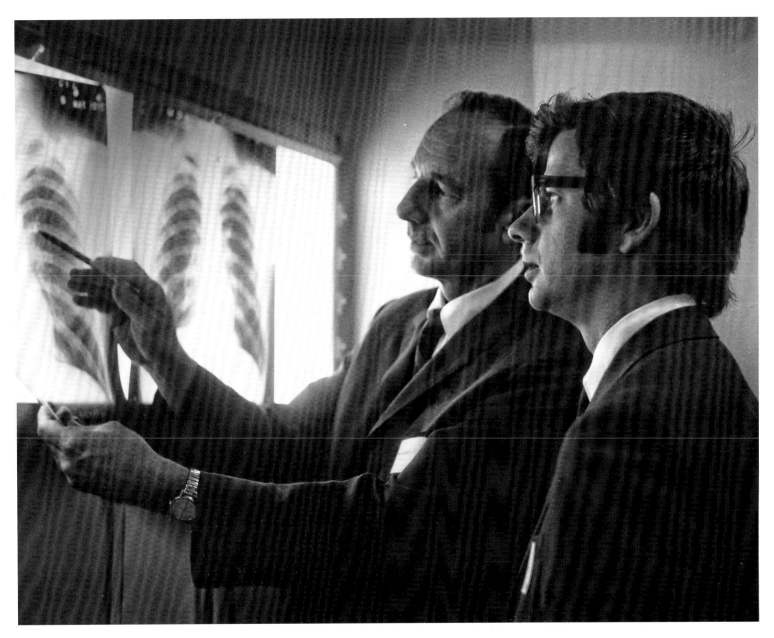

Dr. Paul Roberts (Family Medicine) with resident.

Dr. John Speakman served as Chief of Ophthalmology at Sunnybrook from 1969 until 1988. His leadership at Sunnybrook was cited when he was awarded the Order of Canada. Dr. William Dixon succeeded Speakman as Chief, and stayed for 23 years. He played a significant role in the provincial Eye Bank, organ retrieval, and in establishing the foundation for the Dixon Family Chair in Ophthalmology Research.

Dr. Doug Johnson was appointed the first Chief of Family Medicine. By 1971, the Flemingdon Park Clinic began to function as an outreach site.

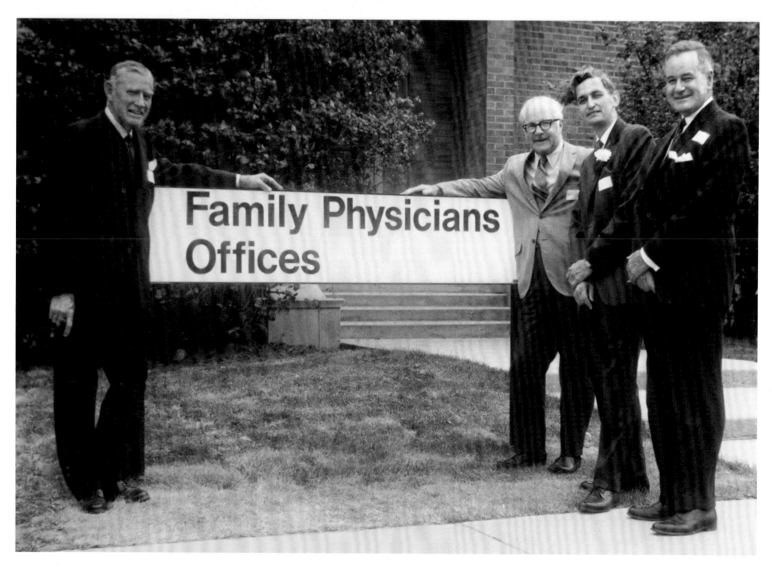

Birth and Growth of a Major Teaching Hospital (1967–1998)

An Emergency service opened in 1971. Within a few years, recruitment to the Emergency Department began to expect fully trained specialists in Emergency Medicine. A helipad was established in 1972, laying one of the foundations for future trauma services.

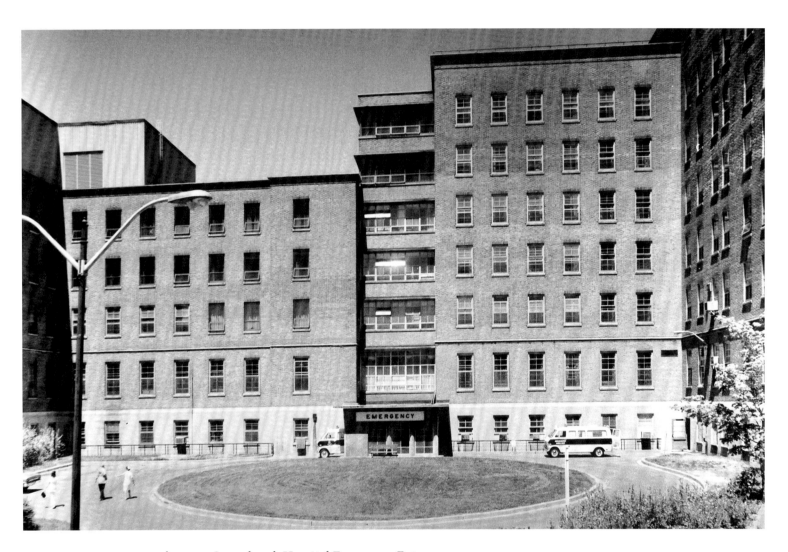

ABOVE: *Sunnybrook Hospital Emergency Entrance*

FACING: *Dr. Douglas Johnson, first Chief of Family Medicine, 1968–88 (second from the right), at the opening of Family Physician Offices.*

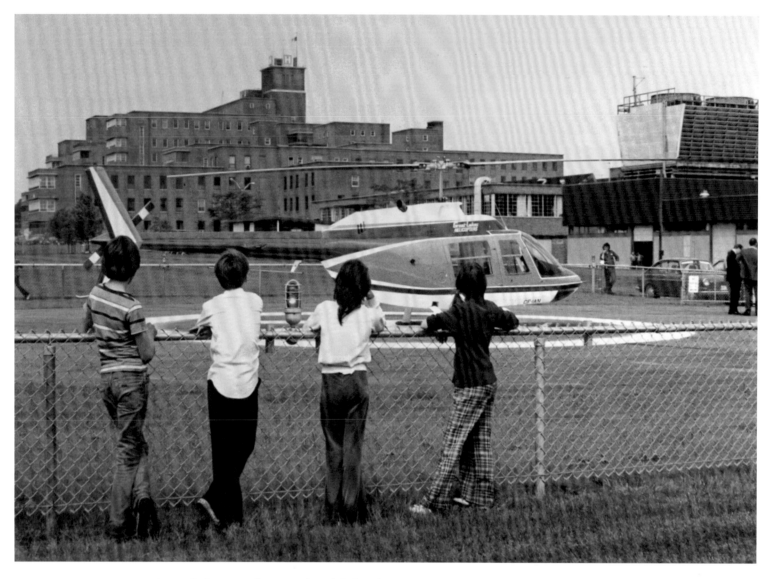

Air ambulance at the Sunnybrook helipad.

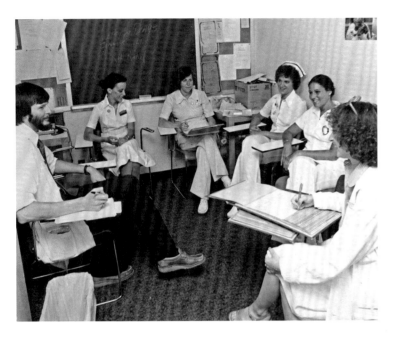

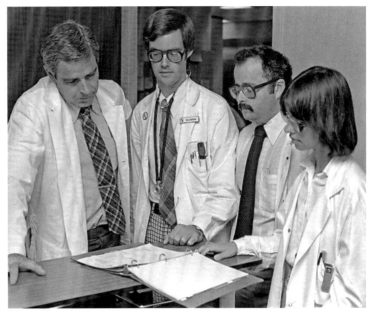

Nursing students (1979).

Drs. Donald Cowan, James Parrish (Resident), David Epstein (Chief Resident), and Anita Rachlis, during teaching rounds.

Dr. Jim Main established the Dentistry department in 1972. Years later, it incorporated the dental services provided to the veterans.

The W.P. Scott Geriatric Day Hospital was founded in 1972, providing a unique outpatient setting for the elderly who needed various kinds of care. By 1988, the Regional Geriatric Program was established, with Dr. Ken Shulman as its founding interim director.

In 1970, a master plan process was initiated, which formally prioritized the capital developments for Sunnybrook Hospital for the next several decades. The initial committee included Dr. J. Kemp Morrison (CEO), Dorothy Wylie (Nursing), Richard Hamilton (Finance), David Shedden (Planning), Dr. Allan Knight (Medicine), Dr. Ian Duncan (Laboratories), and Dr. Al Harrison (Surgery).

Services began to be organized based on patient needs, not on traditional departmental or professional boundaries. This was a precursor to the program-management model that would further evolve in the 1990s. The

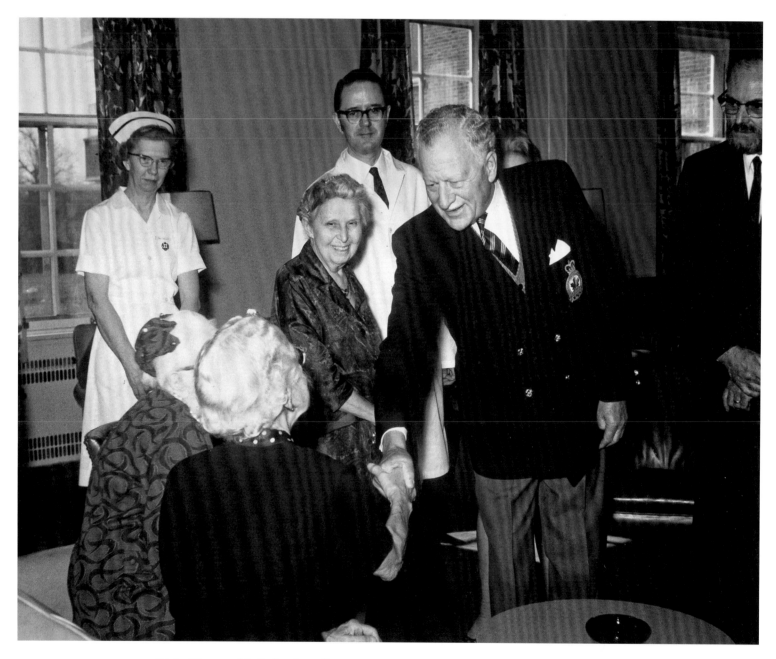

Right Honourable Roland Michener, Governor General of Canada (1967–74) with J. Wallace, Director of Nursing, visiting veterans.

early successes, which now have a long-standing history, included neuro-sciences, led by Dr. Henry Barnett (later awarded the Order of Canada); trauma, led by Dr. Marvin Tile; an approach to musculoskeletal disorders, led by Dr. Hugh Little (Rheumatology) and Dr. Marvin Tile (Orthopaedics); a focus on aging (Dr. Rory Fisher); and Oncology (Drs. Glen Taylor and Al Harrison). Barbara Burke, Director of Nursing, led the development of the nursing manager role, which played a key role in the programs. She also fostered education programs for the staff nurses.

During this era of academic growth, Sunnybrook's role in postgraduate education continued to grow. Saturday morning surgical seminars, led by Dr. Al Harrison, were voluntarily attended by residents and fellows from across Toronto and from as far away as Hamilton, Kingston, and even, on occasion, Ottawa. The lecture theatre is now named Harrison Hall.

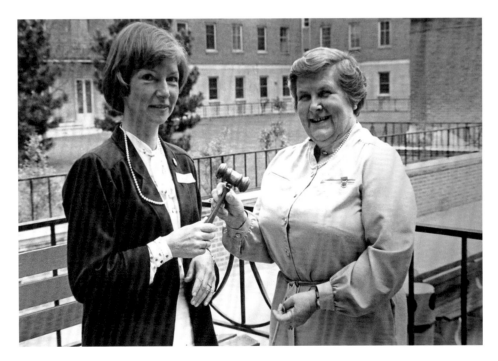

Sue Coate passing the Sunnybrook Hospital Veterans Association gavel to Judy Boynton, 1980.

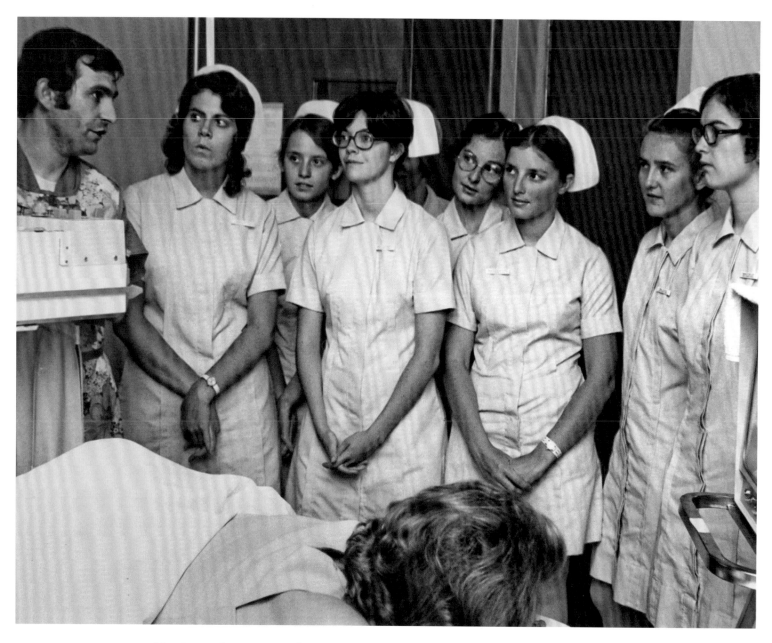

Nursing students on rounds.

In 1973, the physicians at Sunnybrook created the first hospital-wide practice plan. Named the Sunnybrook Hospital University of Toronto Clinic (SHUTC), it contributed significantly to future recruitment. Decades later, it would form the foundation of Sunnybrook's alternate funding plan. Individuals involved in the founding and early growth of SHUTC included Drs. Art Chisholm, Peter Pinkerton, Al Harrison, Ed Kingstone, Hugh Little, and Mr. Jack Morton, the Executive Director.

Also in 1973, Sunnybrook Hospital changed its name to Sunnybrook Medical Centre.

Under the guidance of Drs. Kirk Weber (Anaesthesia) and Glen Taylor (General Surgery) the Surgical Intensive Care Unit moved toward a model in which attending doctors had to possess critical care training. This was an important step toward the future specialization of critical care services.

In 1974, the decades of developing expertise in neurosciences led to the creation of Canada's first Acute Spinal Cord Injury Unit, led by Dr.

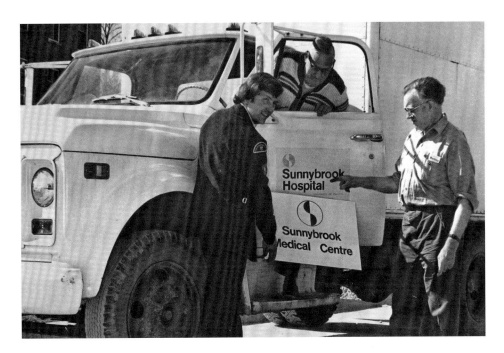

Sunnybrook Hospital becomes Sunnybrook Medical Centre (1973).

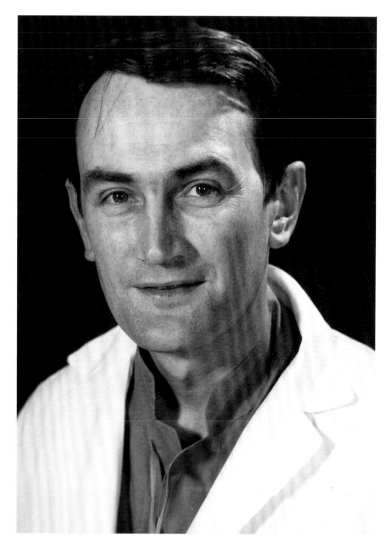

Dr. Kirk Weber, Chief of Anaesthesia (1972–92).

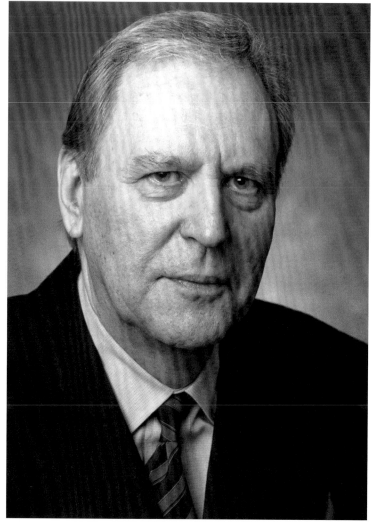

Dr. Alan W. Harrison, Chief of Surgery (1966–67 and 1969–85).

Charles Tator, who was subsequently awarded the Order of Canada for this work. The MacLachlan Stroke Unit, led by neurologist Dr. John Norris and Dr. Vladimir Hachinski, was the first in Canada. Dr. Hachinski became internationally known as a stroke specialist and was later awarded the Order of Canada.

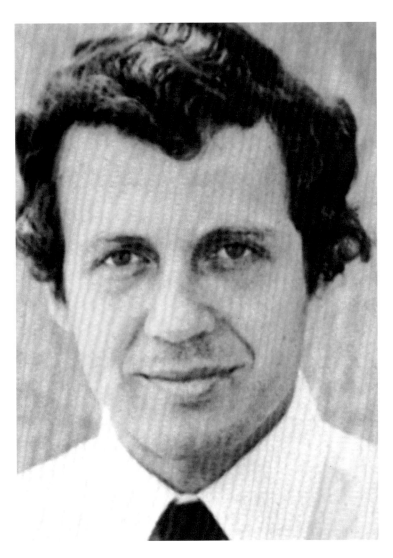

Dr. Bob McMurtry, Chief of Emergency Services (1975–87).

After years of advocacy by individuals such as Dr. Marvin Tile, the Regional Trauma Unit was opened in July 1975. Its first director was Dr. Bob McMurtry. Other key clinical leaders included Dr. Glen Taylor (shock and thoracic injury management), Dr. Michael Schwartz (head injuries), and Dr. Jim Powell (multiple fractures management). Leaders in the care of abdominal injuries included Dr. H.A.B. ("Beans") Miller, Dr. Sherif Hanna, and Dr. Alan Harrison. The Sunnybrook Trauma Program had many associated innovations, such as the "one number to call," based at Sunnybrook, Bandage One helicopter, a program to educate youth about trauma risks (the PARTY Program), and the involvement of Sunnybrook physicians as the base hospital for paramedics. Dr. Tile's clinical expertise, research, and education in the management of pelvic fractures garnered international recognition.

The second half of the 1970s saw the building of the Kilgour Wing (1976), named in honour of the Kilgour family, as a new residence for the veterans at Sunnybrook. The Hees Wing, named in honour of the Honourable George Hees, Minister of Veterans Affairs, opened in 1990 to provide more residential space for veterans.

In the early 1970s, with the radiation therapy resources of the Princess Margaret Hospital (PMH) reaching capacity, a commission was established

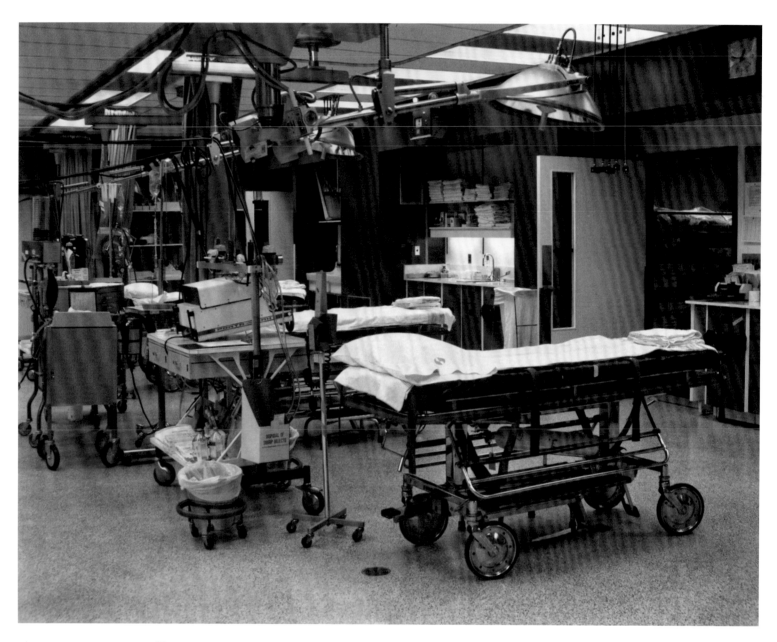

Trauma room.

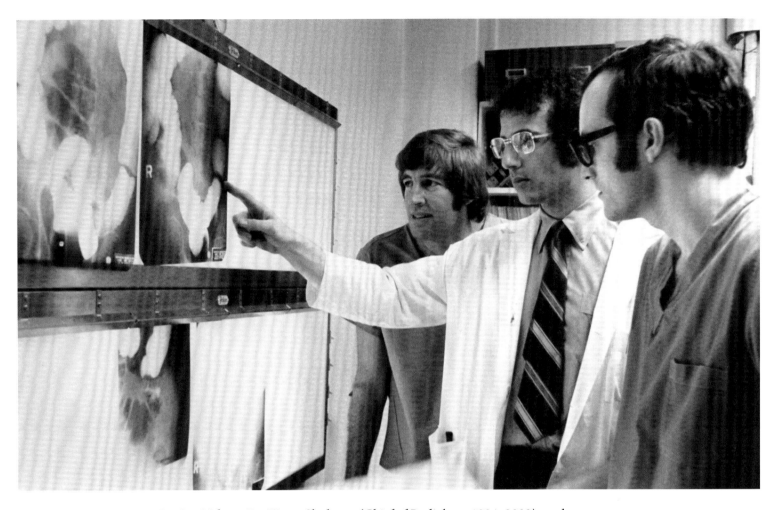

Dr. Jim Nelson, Dr. Harry Shulman (Chief of Radiology, 1984–2003), and Dr. Barry Winning.

to recommend a second site in Toronto for comprehensive cancer care. Sunnybrook was ultimately chosen as the site, largely because of the desire to have a strong research presence in the proposed new centre. Dr. Ray Bush and Dr. Donald Cowan, then at PMH, as well as Dr. K.G.R. Wightman, head of the Ontario Cancer Treatment and Research Foundation, led the planning initiative, which started in earnest in 1974. In the planning stage, the site was named the North Toronto Cancer Centre. The opening of the renamed Toronto-Bayview Regional Cancer Centre, on the site of what had been the Red Cross Lodge, occurred in 1981. Early leadership during this era was provided by Dr. Derek Jenkin (Radiation Oncology) and Dr. David Osoba (Medical Oncology), both of whom were recruited from PMH. Dr. Hugh Barber (Otolaryngology) was an influential force in fostering research

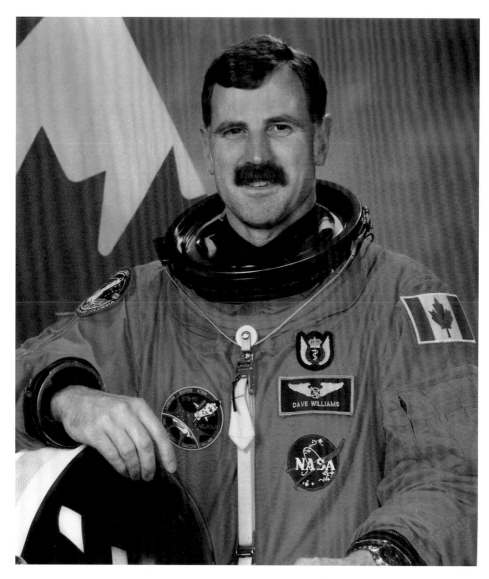

Dr. David Williams, Chief of Emergency Medicine (1992) and a Canadian astronaut.

opportunities for the new cancer centre as well as for the rest of the hospital. Dr. Ralph Gilbert (Otolaryngology) was appointed to the newly created and at the time unique position of Director, Surgical Oncology.

As Sunnybrook entered its second full decade as a teaching hospital, Drs. Kemp Morrison and Martin Barkin, the Hospital Presidents, realized the importance of enhancing the research abilities of the hospital. The First Sunnybrook Fund was launched in 1985 and the Research Wing Building was started in 1987. In 1989, Dr. Mark Henkelman was recruited as the Vice-President, Research. Originally a physicist at the Ontario Cancer Institute (OCI), Dr. Henkelman assembled a group of seven senior imaging scientists from the OCI to join him. This established Sunnybrook as a centre of imaging research excellence within the city. A lasting partnership with Cancer Care Ontario was another legacy of this effort.

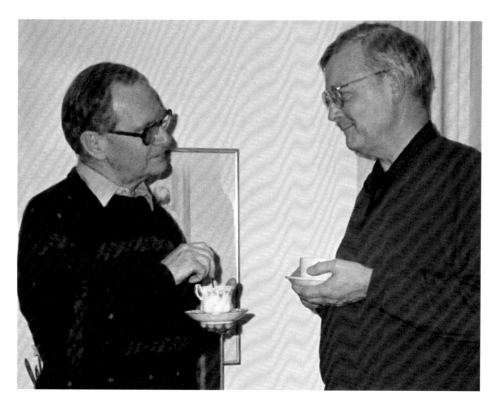

Dr. John Senn (Haematology) and Dr. Hugh Little (Rheumatology).

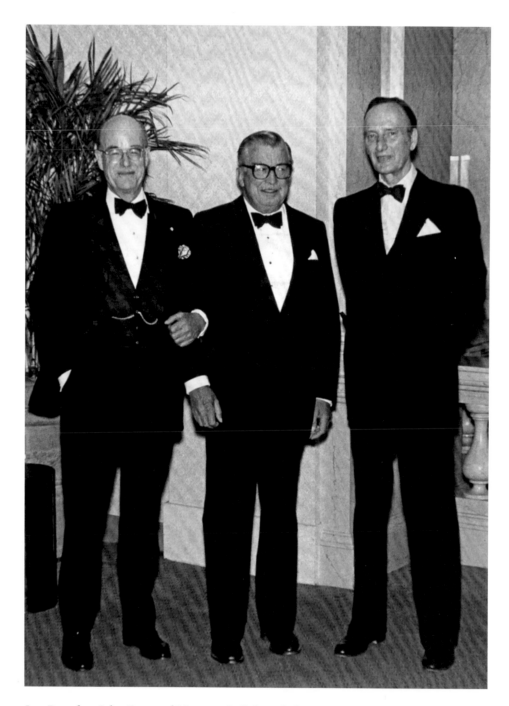

Ian Douglas, John Orr, and Norman Bell, board chairs.

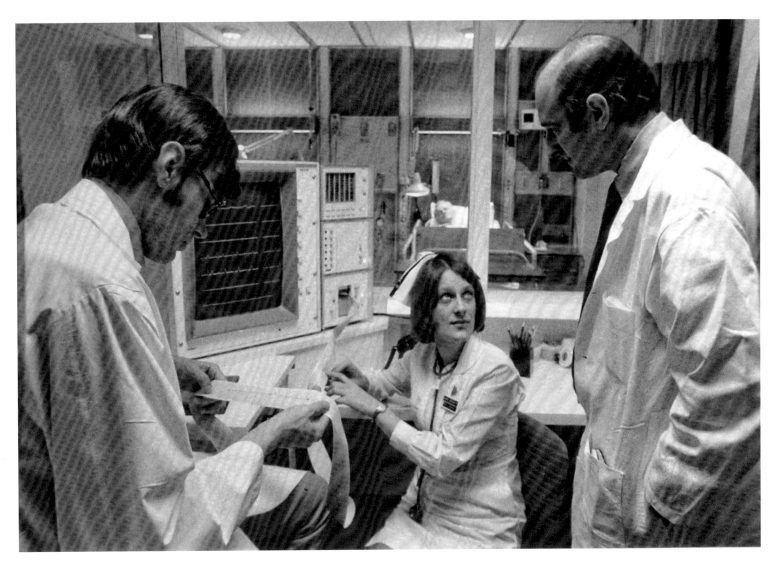

Dr. Vladimir Hachinski (Neurology) and Dr. John Norris (Neurology) in the Stroke Unit.

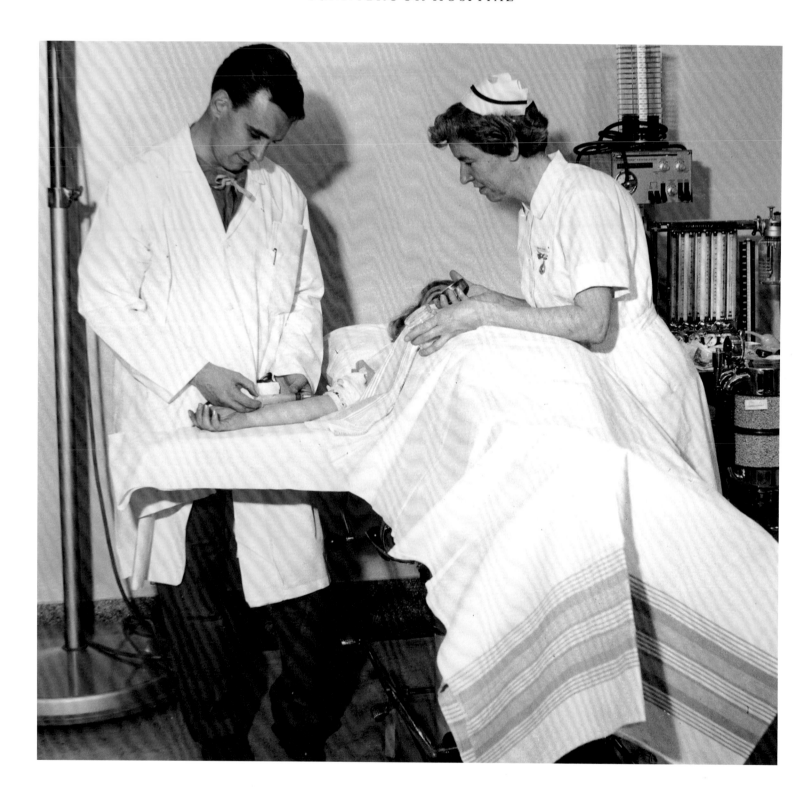

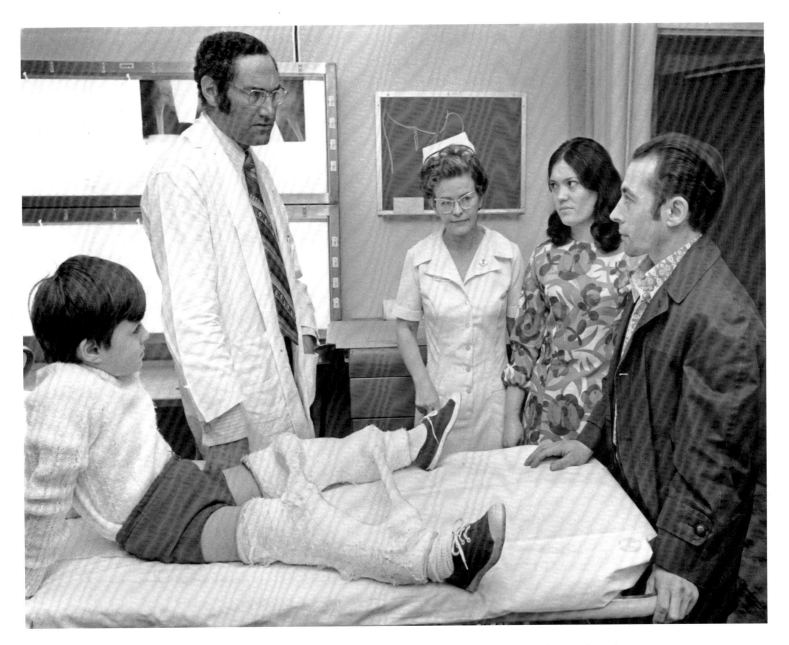

ABOVE: *Dr. Marvin Tile (Chief of Surgery, 1985–96) with Ms. MacPherson (Head Nurse of the Fracture Clinic) and patient with family.*

FACING: *Dr. Glen Taylor (Surgery) with Head Nurse Mary Kane, Emergency Department.*

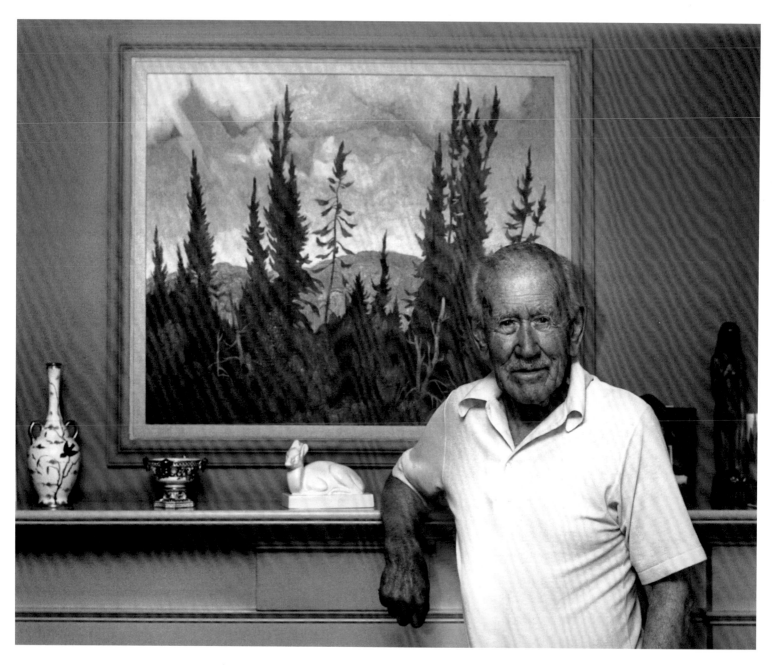

A.J. Casson (1898–1992) Group of Seven artist and resident of Sunnybrook.

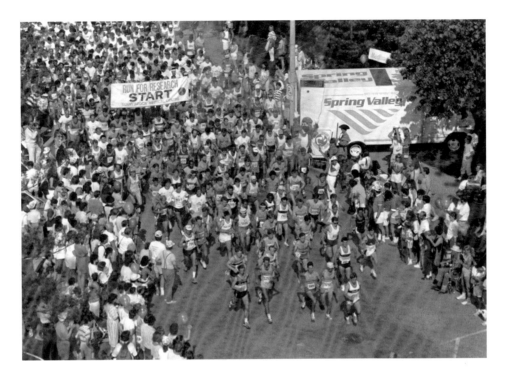

Run for Research.

In 1993, with the hospital's research efforts underway, Peter Ellis, President and CEO, appointed Dr. Peeter Poldre as the hospital's first Vice-President, Health Sciences Education. The early 1990s was a period of curriculum renewal at the Faculty of Medicine. One of the key innovations was the creation of academies, which served as the home base for groups of medical students for at least a two-year period. In 1994, Sunnybrook became the home site of the Boyd Academy of the Faculty of Medicine, named after Dr. William Boyd, former University of Toronto Professor of Pathology and the author of the world's most famous pathology textbook. Dr. Poldre became the Boyd Academy's first Director.

Dr. John Senn was the driving force behind clinical ethics expertise at Sunnybrook. With the assistance of Eric Meslin, Ph.D., Sunnybrook became a key participant in the newly created Joint Centre for Bioethics at the University of Toronto.

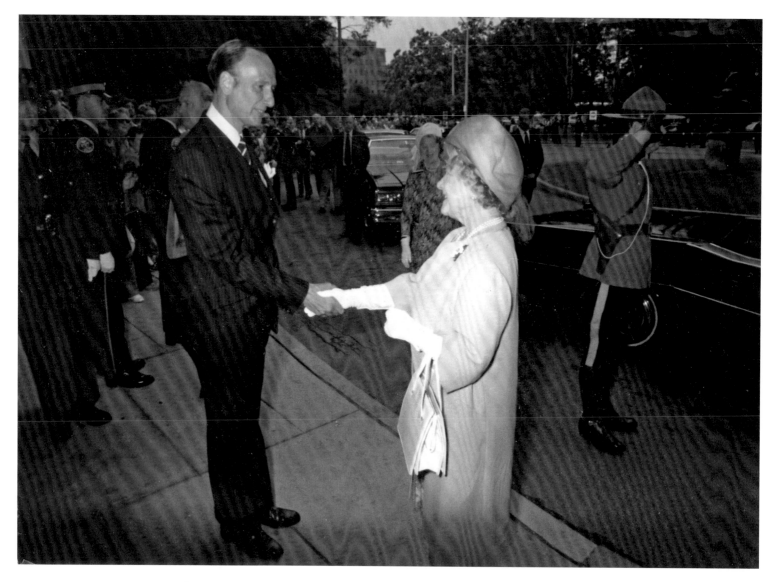

Royal Visit, 1982 — Norman Bell greeting HRH Queen Elizabeth, the Queen Mother.

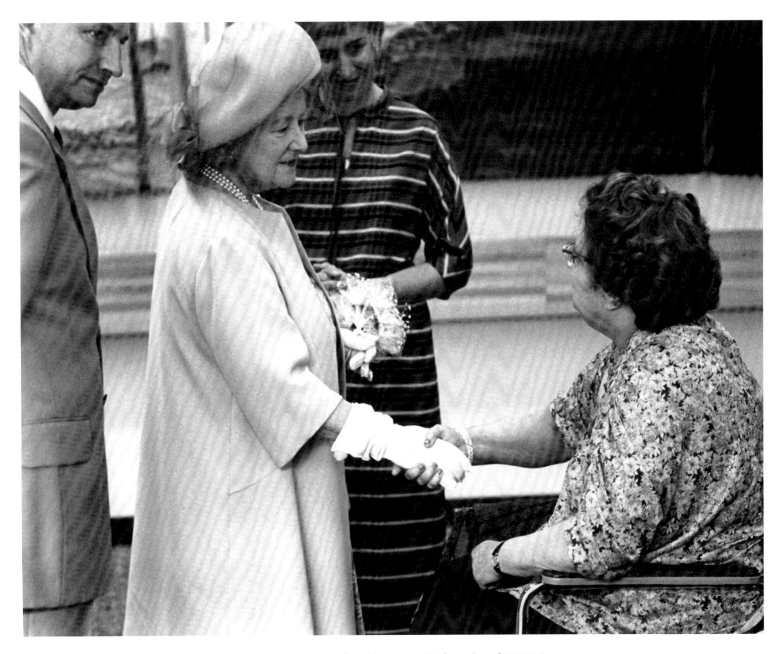

Royal Visit, 1982 — Dr. Rory Fisher (Geriatric Medicine) and HRH Queen Elizabeth, the Queen Mother, greeting a veteran.

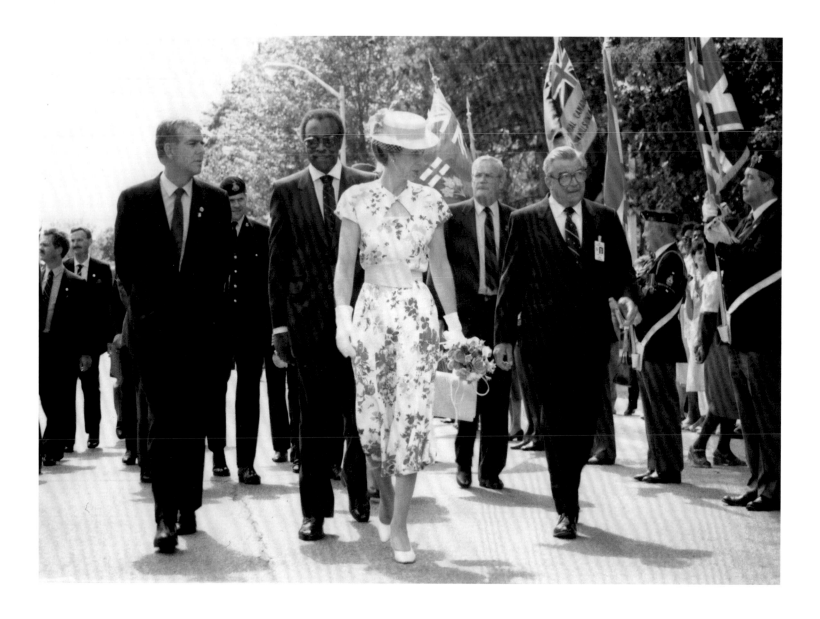

ABOVE: *Royal Visit, 1986 — Left to Right: Right Honourable Lincoln Alexander, Lieutenant Governor of the Province of Ontario; HRH Princess Anne; John Orr, chair, Sunnybrook Board of Trustees.*

FACING: *Royal Visit, 1986 — HRH Princess Anne with Sunnybrook volunteers.*

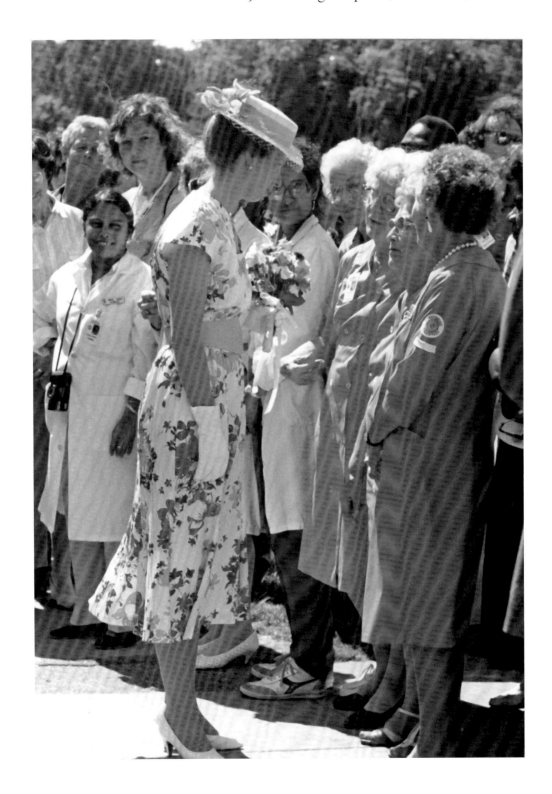

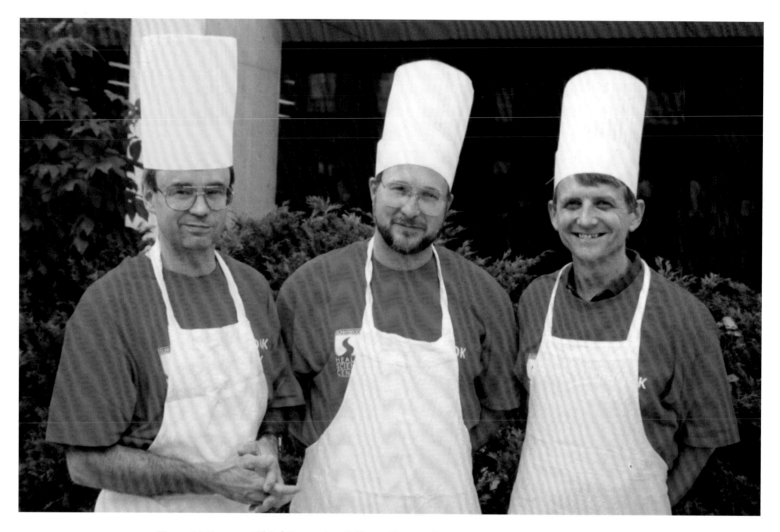

Terry McBurney, Chief Operating Officer, Cancer Centre, Dr. Barry McLellan, Chief of Emergency, and Tom Closson, President and CEO.

In 1992, Dr. Julian Nedzelski began a 10-year term as the University Chair of Otolaryngology. This was the first time that Sunnybrook was the home base for a university chair.

In the late 1980s and early 1990s, under the guidance of Dr. Martin Barkin, and then Peter Ellis and his successor, Mr. Tom Closson, Sunnybrook became known for its program management model of care. Kerry Marshall,

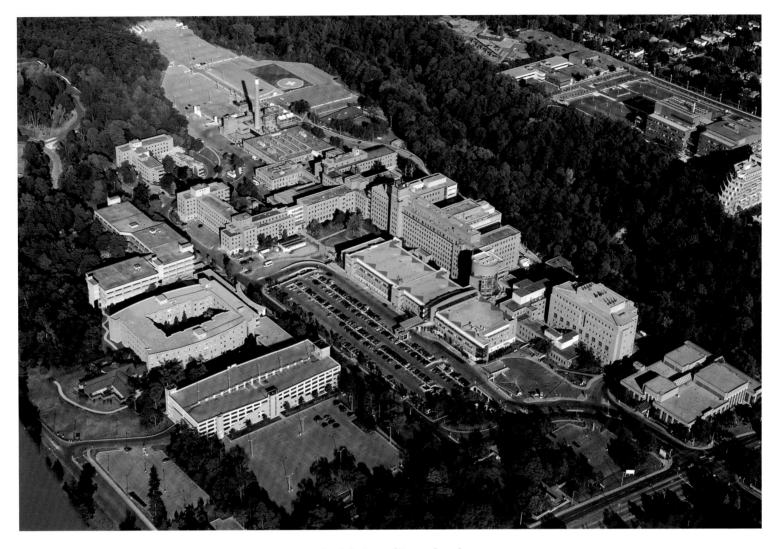

Aerial view of Sunnybrook.

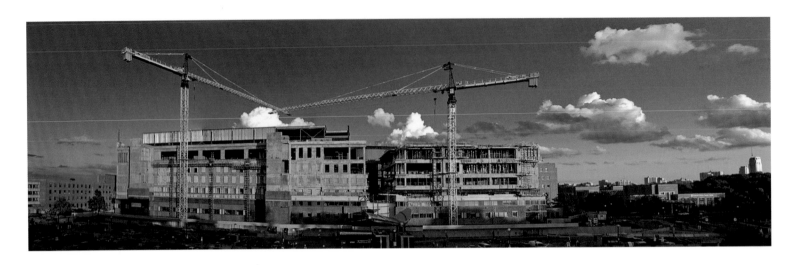

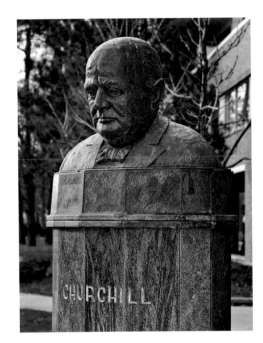

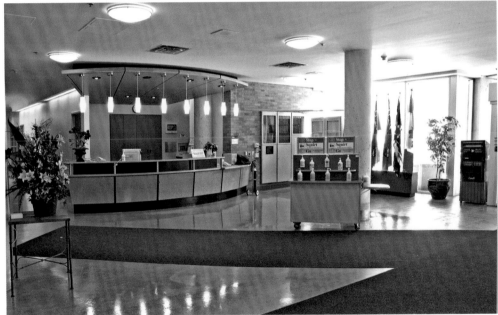

TOP: *Second phase of M-Wing construction underway.*

ABOVE LEFT: *Bronze bust of Winston Churchill (sculptor, Ernest Raab).*
Presented as a gift to the veterans in honour of the fiftieth anniversary of D-Day.

ABOVE RIGHT: *Veterans Centre L-Wing lobby (2010).*

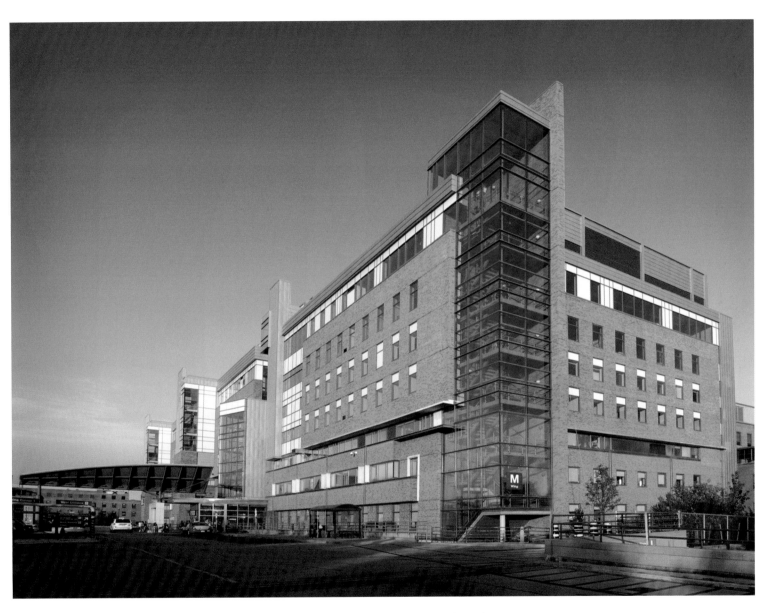

Sunnybrook M-Wing exterior (2009).

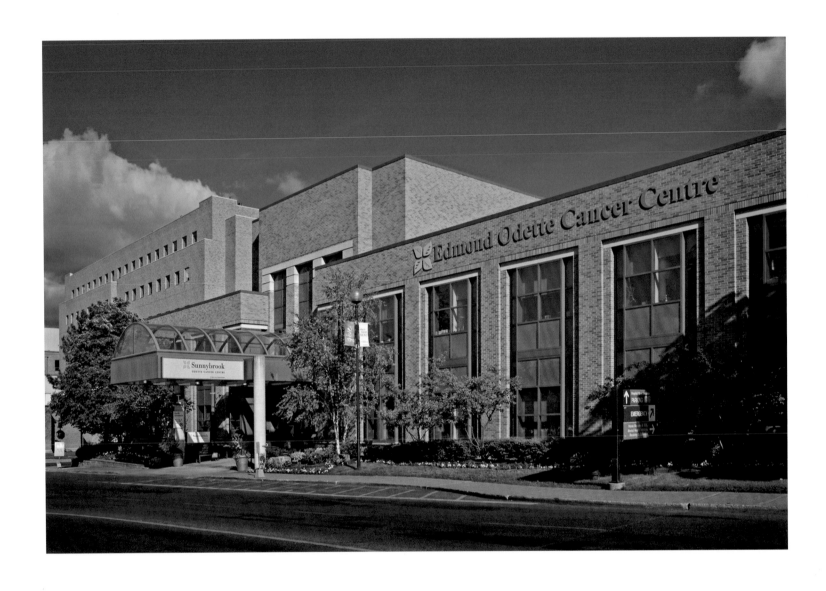

ABOVE: *Edmond Odette Cancer Centre exterior (2009).*

FACING: *Edmond Odette Cancer Centre interior atrium (2009).*

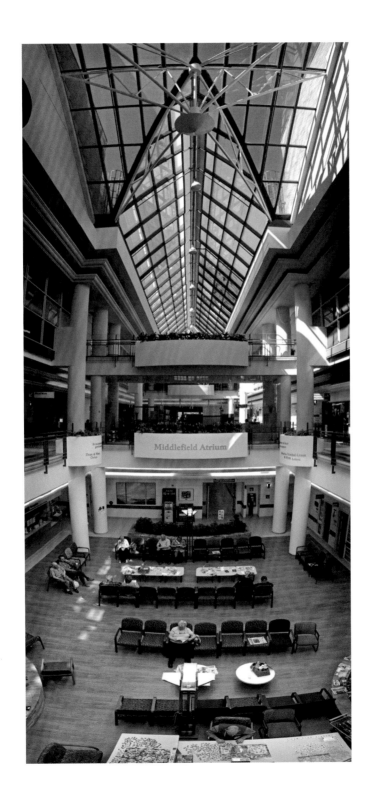

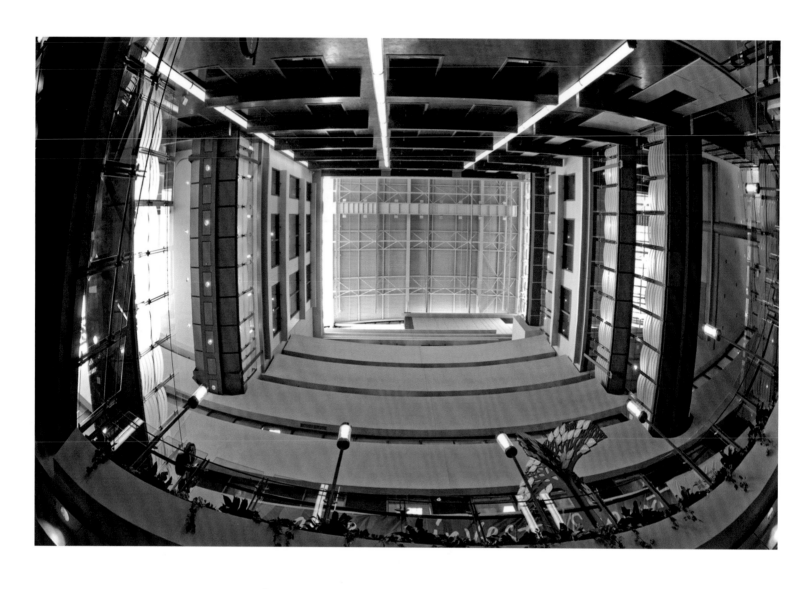

ABOVE AND FACING: *M-Wing main atrium (2010).*

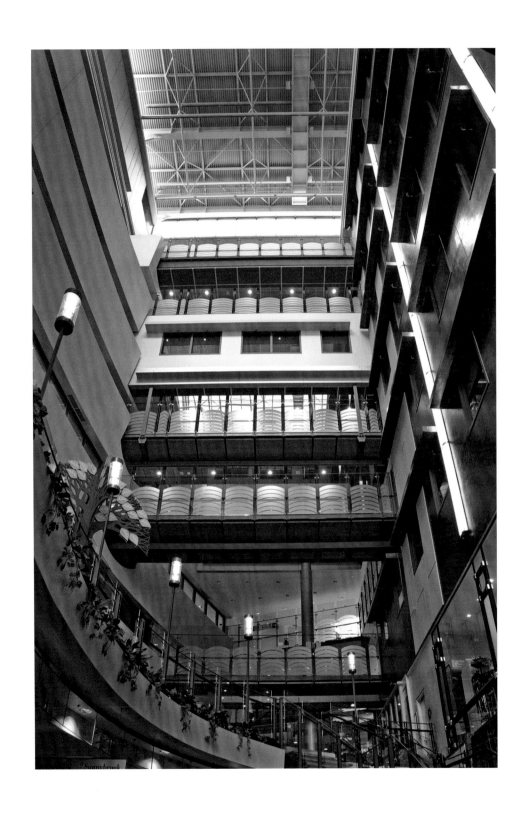

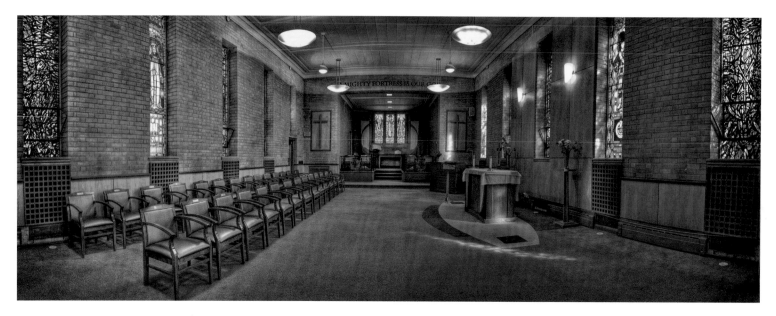

Sunnybrook Chapel.

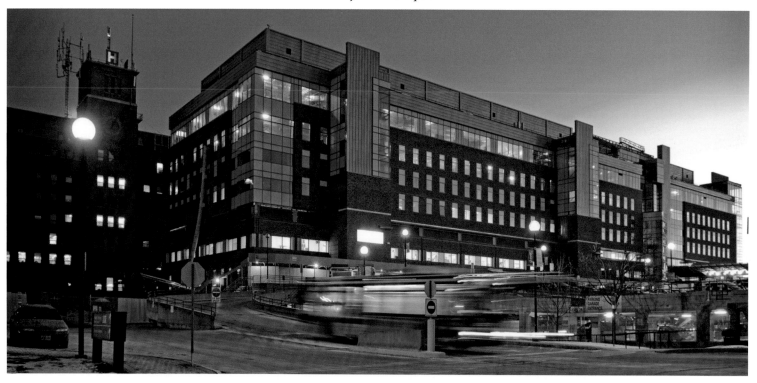

Sunnybrook at night (2009).

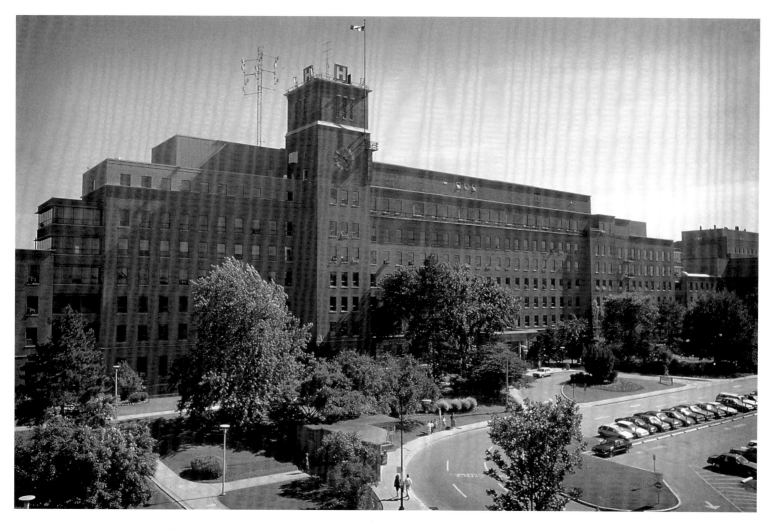

C-Wing exterior view (1993).

Vice-President Nursing (1990–95) and her successor, Gail Mitchell, Ph.D., Director of Nursing (1995–99), led the efforts to include a team-approach philosophy and patient-centered care into the program model. A brief review of the programs follows in the next chapter.

In the 1990s, Sunnybrook's influence reached into outer space. In 1992, Dr. Roberta Bondar became the first Canadian woman and the first

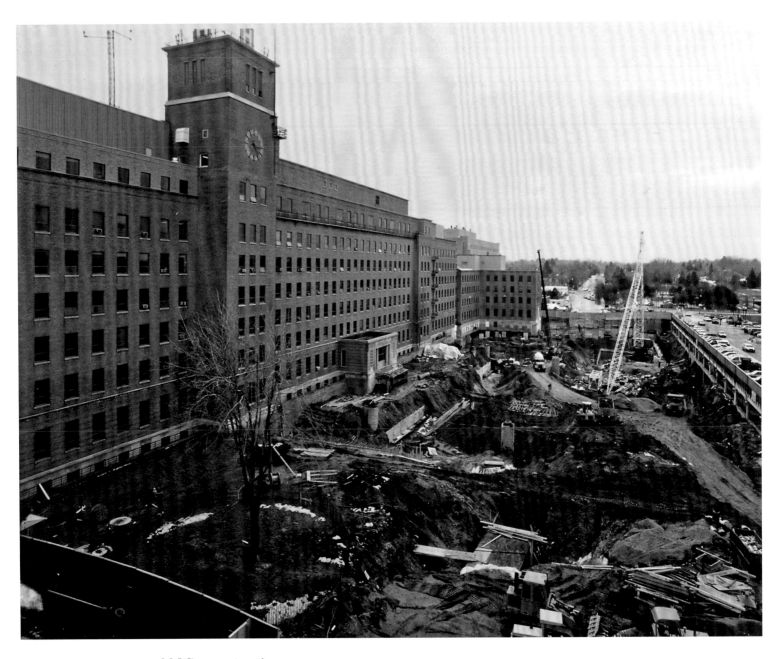

M-Wing construction.

neurologist to travel into space. In 1998, Dr. David Williams, who had been a member of the hospital's Emergency Medicine department, made the first of his two trips into space.

With the building of the Kilgour and the Hees Wings, the Sunnybrook footprint changed dramatically. In 1998, the long-awaited "frontal expansion," M-Wing opened. It included state-of–the-art intensive care units, operating theatres, and an abundance of ambulatory care space for Sunnybrook. But the need for more was just around the corner.

CHAPTER 4

Into the Twenty-First Century

ON JUNE 24, 1998, THE Government of Ontario created an amalgamation of Sunnybrook Health Science Centre, Women's College Hospital, and the Orthopedic & Arthritic Hospital, which was eventually named Sunnybrook and Women's College Health Sciences Centre, or Sunnybrook & Women's for short. Considerable time and effort were spent on the countless issues and details surrounding the governance and management of a large hospital on three geographically different sites. The planned new building to accommodate all the amalgamated services at the Bayview Avenue site was delayed for many years.

Dr. Martin Barkin, a former staff urologist and subsequent President and CEO of Sunnybrook, served as the Chair of the Board of Directors during the first five years of the new hospital. Several key clinical leaders were recruited from other institutions during this transitional period. Dr. Robin Richards, the new Chief of Surgery, was from St. Michael's Hospital. Dr. Jennifer Blake, Chief of Obstetrics & Gynaecology, was from McMaster University. The new Physician-in-Chief, Dr. William Sibbald, came from the University of Western Ontario. In addition to leading the Department of Medicine, he was also vital in establishing the academic prowess of the Department of Critical Care Medicine. Most other department and program leaders who were appointed in this era were from one of the three legacy hospitals.

The amalgamation also affected the academic mandate. The Faculty of Medicine's academies were re-aligned. The academy at Sunnybrook &

Women's became the Peters-Boyd Academy. (In the previous academy structure, Women's College Hospital had been the host site of the Peters Academy. Dr. Vera Peters was a distinguished radiation oncologist.) Dr. Peeter Poldre was chosen to be the Director of the newly named and significantly enlarged Academy. A major boost to the hospital's education mission was a large grant from the McLaughlin Foundation that enabled the building of two state-of-the-art lecture facilities. In 2004, Dr. Leslie Nickell (Family Medicine) became the second academy director for a five-year term. Dr. Catherine Kelly (Women's College Hospital) served as interim director in 2009 until Dr. Mary Anne Cooper (Gastroenterology) assumed the role in 2010.

The new hospital's most senior leadership also saw numerous changes. Shortly after the amalgamation, President and CEO Tom Closson departed. After a transition period, Dr. David McCutcheon was appointed CEO. Subsequently, Leo Steven and Dr. Barry McLellan assumed the Hospital President's role.

Sue VanDeVelde-Coke, Ph.D., became the Chief Nursing and Health Professions Executive in 2004. In close collaboration with the Chief Medical Executives, Dr. Bob Lester (2002–07) followed by Dr. Keith Rose (2008–), a strong leadership model continued. Michael Young and Alison Welch guided the financial health of the hospital. Sam Marafioti led numerous construction efforts as well as information technology. Marilyn Reddick led the Human Resources portfolio during these complicated changes in organizational governance. Craig DuHamel ensured excellent communications to both internal and external stakeholders.

Dr. Michael Julius, an immunologist, became the Vice-President, Research, in 2001. Under his stewardship, the first decade of the 21st century witnessed an exponential growth in Sunnybrook's research enterprise. An important facet of research conducted by Sunnybrook scientists was related to health services research and clinical epidemiology. In 1992, the provincial government had established the Institute for Clinical Evaluative Sciences (ICES), one of Canada's premier health services research institutes. The first CEO of ICES, Dr. David Naylor, was a Sunnybrook specialist in internal medicine who went on to become Dean of the Faculty of Medicine and then President of the University of Toronto.

The Vice-President, Medical Education, Dr. Peeter Poldre, ensured an ongoing focus on the hospital's teaching mandate. Collaboration with the Sunnybrook Foundation, led by Kevin Goldthorp and then Jeff O'Hagan, ensured alignment of hospital needs with fundraising priorities.

The year 2003 was one of the most challenging in the history of many Toronto hospitals, with the onset of Severe Acute Respiratory Syndrome (SARS). Sunnybrook played a significant leadership role both advising the Ministry of Health and Long Term Care on many system-wide facets of care. In addition, clinicians at Sunnybrook cared for the largest number of SARS patients in Canada.

Sunnybrook & Women's ongoing governance and operational challenges caused the provincial government to "demerge" Women's College Hospital from Sunnybrook & Women's, with the exception that the labour & delivery and neonatal care remained under the governance of the new Sunnybrook Health Sciences Centre. The separation took effect on April 1, 2006. Government approval for the building of new facilities for the relocation of perinatal and newborn services allowed for the beginning of the addition of two floors to M-Wing.

Sunnybrook's program management structure evolved to an inter-professional collaborative model, with a dyadic leadership structure in which various key responsibilities are shared between a Medical Program Chief and a Director of Operations.

Dr. Brian Gilbert, from Mt. Sinai Hospital, came in 1995 to lead the Heart Program. Earlier, in 1989, cardiac surgery had begun at Sunnybrook, under the leadership of Dr. Bernard Goldman. The program evolved over the decade into the Schulich Heart Centre. Dr. Robert Maggisano (Vascular surgery) dedicated enormous energies into the development and success of endovascular aortic repair (EVAR). The Maggisano Family Chair in Vascular Surgery was created in 2010. Dr. Bradley Strauss (Cardiology) became the Schulich Heart Centre Program Chief in 2010. He also held the Reichmann Chair in Cardiovascular Sciences since 2006.

Jane DeLacy and Susan Michaud were the Directors of Operations for the Heart Program.

A significant addition to the Trauma Program was the relocation of the Ross Tilley Burn Unit, under the leadership of Dr. Joel Fish, from The Wellesley Hospital to Sunnybrook in 2000. The Trauma Program continued as Canada's premier service, with Drs. Barry McLellan, Fred Brenneman, and Gordon Rubenfeld providing medical leadership from 1991 to the present and Debra Carew more recently serving as Director of Operations.

In 2000, Wellspring, a support centre for cancer patients, opened on the Sunnybrook campus. Dr. Sherif Hanna became the Director of Surgical Oncology in 2001. In 2007, he was named the inaugural Hanna Family Chair in Surgical Oncology. A province-wide reorganization of Cancer Care Ontario led to the integration of the renamed Toronto-Sunnybrook Regional Cancer Centre into Sunnybrook in 2004. Several years later, it was named the Odette Cancer Centre. Drs. Derek Jenkin, Ken Shumak, Carol Sawka, and Linda Rabeneck guided the centre during this era, with the collaboration of Yvette Matyas, the Director of Operations. The combined ambulatory and inpatient resources made the Cancer Centre the second largest in Canada.

The combined orthopaedic surgery resources from the Orthopaedic & Arthritic Hospital and Sunnybrook amalgamation created the largest division of orthopaedic surgery in Canada. The Musculo-Skeletal Program, later named the Holland Program, was led initially by Dr. John Cameron. He was succeeded by Dr. Hans Kreder, who also assumed the Marvin Tile Chair in Orthopedic Surgery. Anne Marie MacLeod was the Director of Operations.

In the early 1990s, Sunnybrook's Mental Health Program consisted largely of the Department of Psychiatry. In the early 2000s, under the leadership of Dr. Ken Shulman, the former Chief of Psychiatry, the Neurosciences Program evolved to include elements of Neurology, Geriatric medicine, Neuropathology, and Neurosurgery. It was later renamed the Brain Sciences Program, with Lois Fillion as the Director of Operations. Dr. Shulman was also the inaugural Lewar Chair in Geriatric Psychiatry (2002). The program is home to noted clinician-scientists such as Drs. Sandra Black (cognitive neurosciences) and Anthony Levitt (mood disorders).

As the veterans aged, Sunnybrook staff developed special expertise in managing elderly patients. In 2001, the Dorothy Macham Home opened, providing unique care for the special needs of veterans who have challenging behaviours due to dementia. The Aging Program, initially led by Dr. Heather MacDonald and later by Dr. Jocelyn Charles and Dorothy Ferguson, played an integral role in the care of the veterans who reside in K and L Wings. The program was later renamed the Veterans and Community Program to reflect this special role. K and L Wing were formally renamed as the Sunnybrook Veterans Centre.

The creation of Sunnybrook & Women's in 1998 led to the establishment of the Perinatal & Gynecology Program, which included a neonatal intensive care unit. Under the leadership of Dr. Andrew Shennan and Jo Watson (Ph.D.), the program functioned on an interim basis at 76 Grenville Street while new facilities were being built at the Sunnybrook campus. The program changed its name to the Women & Babies Program in 2009 and relocated to 2075 Bayview Avenue on September 12, 2010.

During the decade, Sunnybrook developed expertise in quality and patient safety. Dr. William Geerts (Respirology) is a world-renowned authority on the prevention of venous thromboembolic disease and authored guidelines that were used at Sunnybrook and internationally. Sunnybrook, partnering with the Hospital for Sick Children, became the host site for the University of Toronto Centre for Patient Safety, lead by two Sunnybrook Internal Medicine specialists, Dr. Kaveh Shojania (Director) and Dr. Edward Etchells (Associate Director).

At the end of the decade, three Sunnybrook surgeons were awarded the Order of Canada, in recognition of their contributions to Canadian medicine. They included Dr. Joseph Schatzker (Orthopaedics), Dr. Marvin Tile (Orthopaedics), and Dr. Bernard Goldman (Cardiac surgery).

Sunnybrook's history began with its dedication to serving the needs of Canada's war veterans. Excellence in patient care, education, and research enriched the care of our veterans and laid the foundation for Sunnybrook's added roles of service to the communities it now serves. Sunnybrook's future will continue to unfold with its commitment to achieving its vision to invent the future of health care.

Acknowledgements and Apologies

THE GENEROUS DONATION BY THE Raab family has made this book possible. The contribution of Veterans Affairs Canada is also gratefully acknowledged. Both the editorial committee and the future readers of the book express their gratitude.

It has been a privilege to work with a superb volunteer editorial committee. Their tireless efforts were led by the remarkable spirit and determination of Marian Lorenz, whose administrative career in various positions at Sunnybrook began in 1954 and lasted 50 years until her retirement in 2004. She has continued to assist with many other projects requiring a historical perspective, such as this book. Other editorial committee members include Archivist Phil Gold, Dr. Alan Harrison, Dr. Donald Cowan, Dr. Marvin Tile, Sally Fur, Bernice Baumgart, and Dale Roddick, our photography expert.

Many others contributed ideas, photos, verification of details, and, most importantly, inspiration and encouragement. In alphabetical order, thanks are owed to: Harold Averill (University of Toronto Archives); Irma Coucill (artist); Norman Bell; Dr. Brian Cuthbertson; Dr. William Dixon; Craig DuHamel, Ph.D.; Dr. Gil Faclier; Kevin Goldthorp; Trudy Hueper; Dr. Kevin Imrie; Dr. Michael Julius; Dr. Robert Lester; Derek Little; Sam Marafioti; Dr. Barry McLellan; Doug Nicholson; Jeff O'Hagan; Ileana Rontea; Dr. Harry Shulman; Dr. Ken Shulman; and Dr. Susan Sutherland.

The four brief chapters are intended as a factual introduction of the key events in each era, allowing the photographs to be understood in the context of what was happening at Sunnybrook.

The accompanying lists of hospital leaders, specifically Superintendents, Presidents and Chief Executive Officers, Chairs and Members of the Boards of Trustees and Directors, and Clinical Department Chiefs reflect the highest levels of leadership over the past decades.

In no way can this book do justice to the many thousands of doctors, nurses, health professionals, employees, volunteers, students, and researchers who have collectively saved and improved the lives of tens of thousands of patients and veterans throughout the history of the hospital. It is fervently hoped that others in future narratives will capture those many elements.

PEETER A. POLDRE, M.D.
EDITOR

Hospital Leaders

Colonel K. Hollis —
Superintendent 1943–1949

B.M. Griffin —
Superintendent 1949

Dr. C. McLeod —
Superintendent 1950–1961

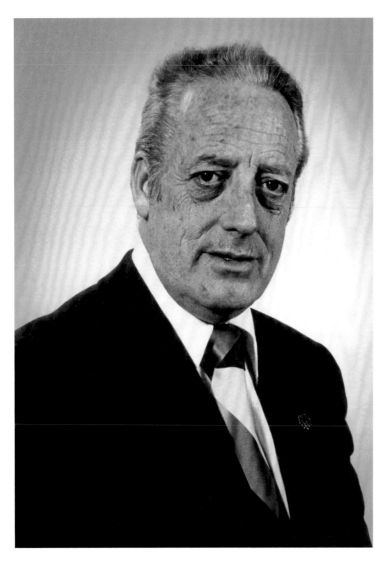

Dr. J.K. Morrison —
Superintendent 1962-1966 / President 1966–1983

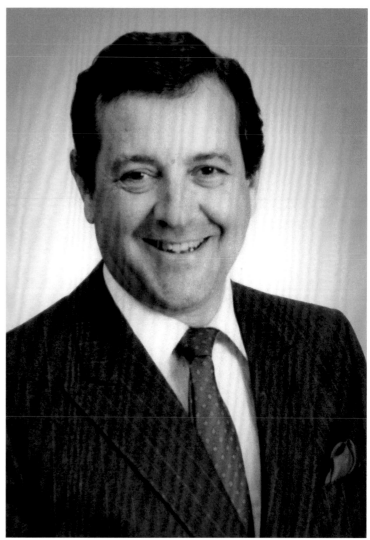

Dr. M. Barkin —
President and Chief Executive Officer 1984–1987

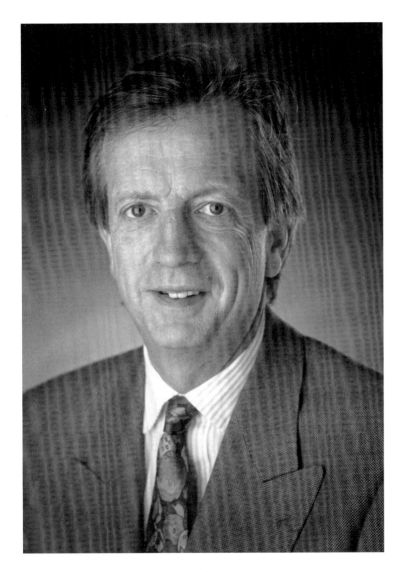

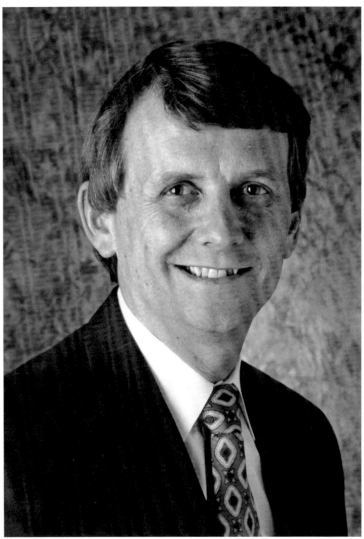

P. Ellis —
President and Chief Executive Officer 1987–1995

T. Closson —
President and Chief Executive Officer 1995–1998

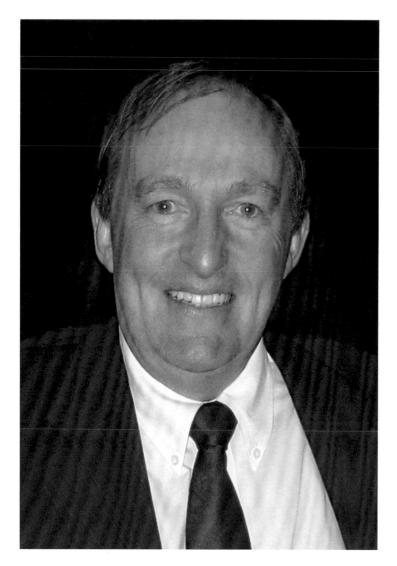

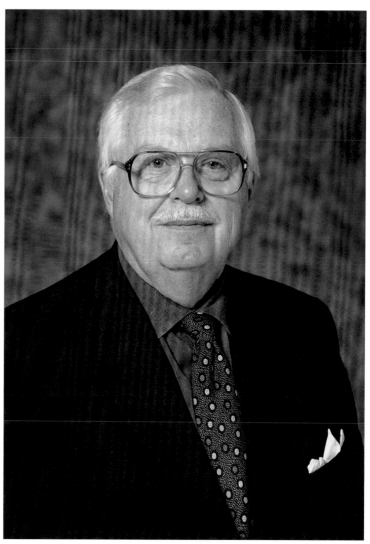

Dr. D. McCutcheon —
President and Chief Executive Officer 1999–2001

A.R. Thorfinnson —
President and Chief Executive Officer 2001–2002

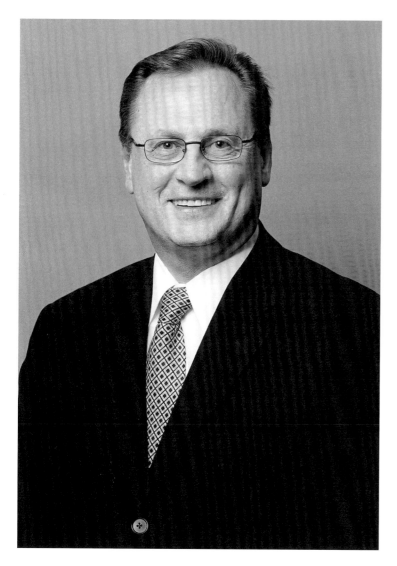

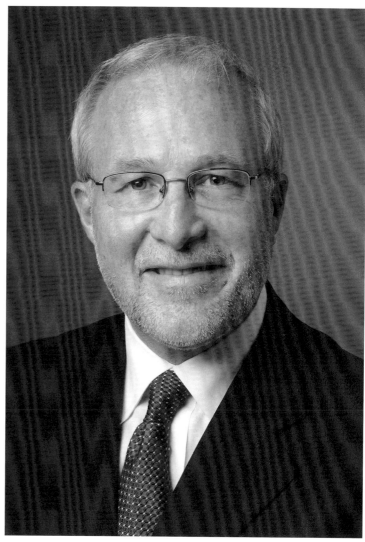

L. Steven —
President and Chief Executive Officer 2002–2007

Dr. B.A. McLellan —
President and Chief Executive Officer 2007–Present

Members of the Board of Trustees — 1960s

Members of the Board of Trustees — 1970s

Members of the Board of Trustees —
1980s

Members of the Board of Trustees — 1990s

Chairs of the Board of Directors

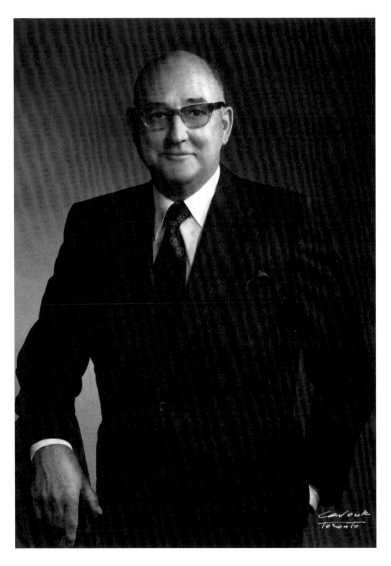

B.H. Rieger (1966–1972)

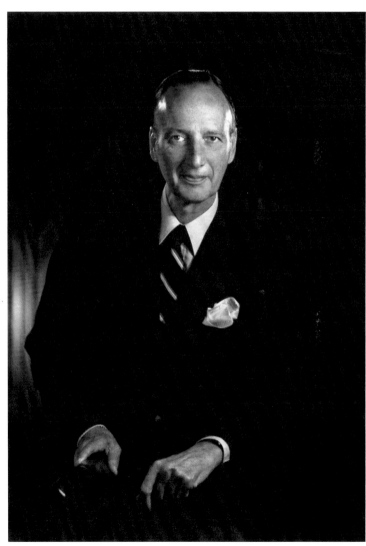

N.B. Bell (1972–1982)

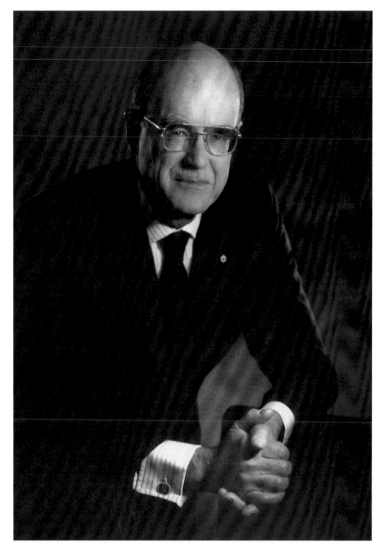

I. Douglas, Q.C. (1982–1985)

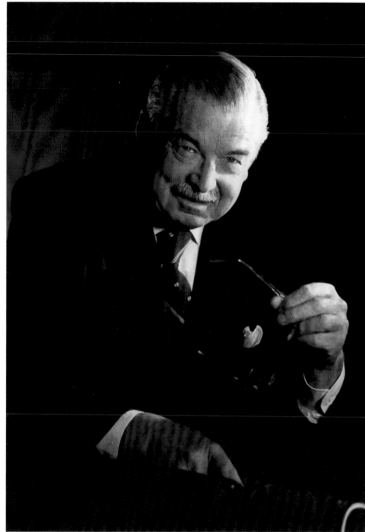

J.A. Orr (1985–1987)

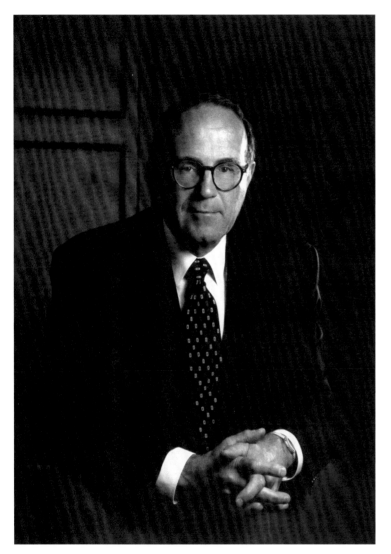

J.M.G. Scott (1987–1992)

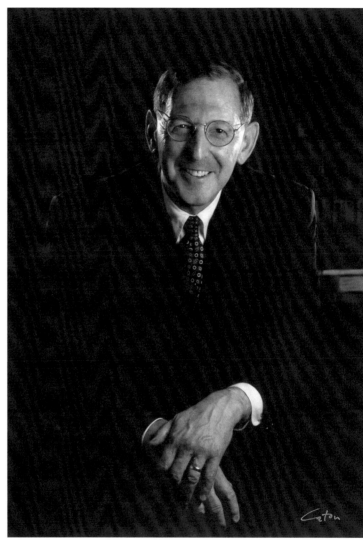

A. Beutel (1992–1995)

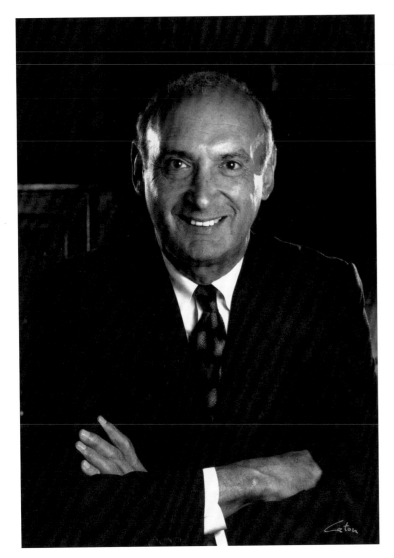

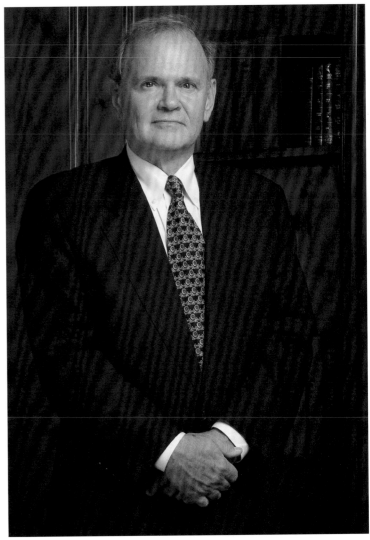

T. Brent (1995–1998)

Dr. A. Aberman (1998)

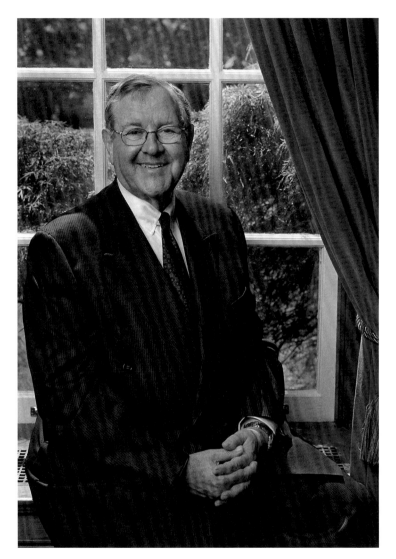

Dr. M. Barkin (1998–2003)

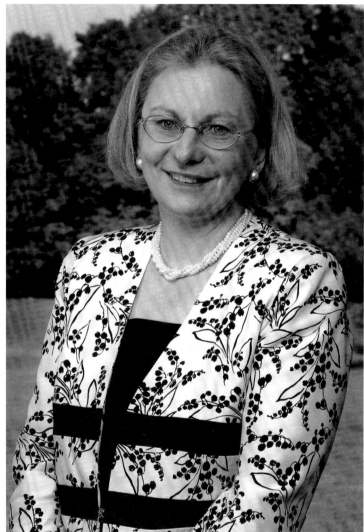

V. McLaughlin (2003–2007)

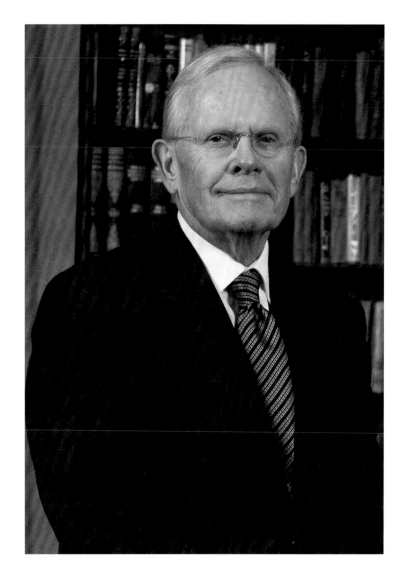

D.A. Leslie (2007–)

Clinical Department Chiefs
1946–2010

SURGERY

J.A. MacFarlane	1946–1959
C. Aberhart	1959–1966
A.W. Harrison	1966–1967*
A.W. Farmer	1966–1969
A.W. Harrison	1969–1985
M. Tile	1985–1996
J.D. Beatty	1996–1999
B. Goldman	1999–2001*
R. Richards	2001–

MEDICINE

R.I. Macdonald	1947–1966
D. MacKenzie	1966*
J.F. Paterson	1966–1974
A. Knight	1974*
D.H. Cowan	1974–1986
A.H. Little	1986–1988*
D.K. Roncari	1988–1993

J. Edmeads	1993–2000
W. Sibbald	2000–2006
A. Aberman	2006–2007*
W. Levinson	2007–2009
K. Imrie	2009–

PHYSICAL MEDICINE AND REHABILITATION

G.A. Lawson	1947–1967
C.M. Godfrey	1967–1971*
K.A. Sowden	1971–1986
P.S. Tepperman	1986–1987
J.H. Somerville	1987–1989

PATHOLOGY (ANATOMIC)

B. Blanchard	1947–1961
J. Barry	1961–1968
B. Cruickshank	1968–1983
S.N. Huang	1984–1994
I. Dube	1994–2000
W. Hanna	2000–2010
M. Khalifa	2010–

MICROBIOLOGY

M. Ross	1947–1966
I. Duncan	1967–1992
A. Simor	1993–

ANAESTHESIA

D. Campbell	1948–1953
J.M. Shapley	1955–1968
A. Noble	1968–1971
R.K. Weber	1972–1992
J.H. Devitt	1992–2000
D. Penning	2000–2001
G. Faclier	2001–

OTOLARYNGOLOGY

C. Rae	1948–1966
P.E. Ireland	1966–1969
H.O. Barber	1969–1986
J. Nedzelski	1986–2007
J. Chen	2007–

PSYCHIATRY

F. Van Nostrand	1948–1969
W. Boothroyd	1969–1971
E. Kingstone	1971–1977
R.F. Billings	1977–1978
V. Rakoff	1978–1980
S. Levine	1981–1991
K. Shulman	1992–2001
A. Levitt	2001–

RADIOLOGY/MEDICAL IMAGING

D. Burke	1949–1957
K. Hodge	1958–1961
J.N. Harvie	1962–1968
D.L. McRae	1968–1977
J.E. Campbell	1977–1984
H. Shulman	1984–2003
A. Moody	2003–

CRITICAL CARE MEDICINE
(FORMERLY SURGICAL INTENSIVE CARE UNIT)

A.W. Harrison	1959–1971
R.K. Weber	1971–1980
S.R. Reid	1980–1991
R.F. McLean	1991–1998
J.H. Devitt	1998–1999
P. Murphy	1999–2001
C. Guest	2001–2003
A. Aberman	2003–2004*
W. Sibbald	2004–2006
R. Fowler	2006–2009*
B. Cuthbertson	2009–

BIOCHEMISTRY

A. Malkin	1962–1990

LABORATORY HAEMATOLOGY

P. Pinkerton   1967–1999

LABORATORY MEDICINE

P. Pinkerton   1990–1999

CLINICAL PATHOLOGY

M. Reis   2000–

FAMILY MEDICINE

D.H. Johnson	1968–1988
P. Norton	1988–1993
J.R. Gilbert	1994–1999
J. Ruderman	2000–2009
J. Charles	2009–

OPHTHALMOLOGY

J.C. McCulloch	1966*
J.S. Speakman	1967–1988
W. Dixon	1987–2010
P. Kertes	2010–

SUNNYBROOK HOSPITAL

OBSTETRICS & GYNAECOLOGY

J. Harkins	1969–1971
R.H. Wesley	1971–1983
P.L. Chan	1983–1993
M. Shier	1993–2000
J. Blake	2000–

DENTISTRY

J. Main	1972–2003
J. Tsafaroff (veterans)	1980–1993
S. Sutherland	2003–

EXTENDED CARE

R.H. Fisher	1973–1992

EMERGENCY

R. McMurtry	1975–1987
R. Stewart	1988–1989
B. McLellan	1989–1992
D. Williams	1992*
A. McCallum	1993–1998
A. McDonald	2000–2005
P. Hawkins	2005–2006*
J. Tyberg	2006–

RADIATION ONCOLOGY

D. Jenkin	1980–1988
A. Dembo	1988–1991
G.M. Thomas	1991–2001
S. Wong	2002–

NEWBORN & DEVELOPMENTAL PAEDIATRICS

M. Dunn	2001–2009
A. Moore	2009–2010*
S. Lee	2010–

* indicates an acting or interim role

Sunnybrook Foundation Chairs

N. Bell (1979–1981)

Colonel F. McEachren (1981–1982)

A. Russell (1982–1984)

Brigadier P. Cameron (1984–1990)

M. Sabia (1990–1992)

B.V. Kelly (1992–1994)

T.I. Ronald (1994–1997)

Dr. M. Tile (1997–2002)

H.G. Emerson (2002–2003)

H. Barry (2003–2004)

T. O'Sullivan (2004–2006)

J. Tory (2006–2008)

Dr. S. Cooper (2008–2010)

P. Dellelce (2010–)

Sunnybrook Foundation
Board of Directors —
1979–2010

SUNNYBROOK HOSPITAL

J.M. Horgan

G. Homer

D. Jackson

H. Jannson

M.L. Jones

Dr. M. Julius

V. Kanwar

A.O. Kaye

B.V. Kelly

J. Kennedy

T. Kennedy

S. Kerr

M. Koerner

S. Koerner

D. Lam

J.R. LeMesurier

D. Leslie

Dr. J. Leyerle

R. Ling

W. Livingston

A. Lopes

P. Lounsbery

W.C. Lovas

S. Mabro

S. Marshall

L. McCaughey

Col. F. McEachren

B. McGrath

V. McLaughlin

Dr. B. McLellan

W. Mcnee

J. McSherry

A. Mingay

B. Moore

F. Morneau Sr.

Dr. K. Ng

C. Orr

T. O'Sullivan

L. Pagnutti

B. Pope

V. Pringle

E. Pun

A. Reichmann

H. Reid

Dr. R. Richards

J. Robitaille

T.I. Ronald

D. Roncari

R.J. Rosen

R. Ross

A. Russell

M. Sabia

G. Schmid

D. Scott

J.M. Scott

P. Sharpe

J. Sherrington

Dr. K. Shulman

G. Sievwright

N. Nanji-Simard

J. Tanenbaum

J. Temerty

J. Thompson

Dr. M. Tile

S. Tile

E. Tory

J. Tory

A. Tse

J. Underwood

J. Vivash

L. Ward

P. Webb

M. Wekerle

J. Wetmore

M. Wright